Praise for *Rise and Shine*

"Simon Lewis's vivid account of his recovery should be a guidebook for all disabled individuals and their families. His disciplines directly mirror the training of an athlete: 'Go into battle prepared to win.'"
—MIKE UTLEY, former Detroit Lion and President of the Mike Utley Foundation

"A beautiful account of a tragic experience. Simon's courage, indefatigability, and pure humanity shine through every grueling step of his journey back from the rim of death. As he recounts each courageous and agonizing step, he shows us that, at the end of the day, healing is truly a reweaving of body, mind, and spirit. Thank you, Simon, for sharing your arduous, light-filled path with us. You give us hope."
—DAPHNE ROSE KINGMA, author of
Coming Apart: Why Relationships End and How to Live through the Ending of Yours

"Simon Lewis has transformed his own personal tragedy and pain following a horrific car accident by documenting his adjustment to the double challenge of losing his wife and discovering his own disabilities. His autobiography will inspire other neurological patients and their families and give them hope."
—SIMON BARON-COHEN, Professor of Developmental Psychopathology, Cambridge University

"Despite suffering a terrible accident and the sad loss of his wife, Simon Lewis found dignity, bravery, and strength in his magnificent recovery. I found it inspiring and uplifting to read his words, which are beautifully written. Lewis's journey and experience will, I am sure, give hope to many people like myself who are recovering from head and brain injuries, as well as to their families. *Rise and Shine* is a story of courage and determination, and it offers valuable insights into the world of those who suffer brain injuries."
—ASAD AHMAD, presenter and reporter,
BBC London News

Published by: Santa Monica Press LLC
P.O. Box 1076
Santa Monica, CA 90406-1076
1-800-784-9553
www.santamonicapress.com
books@santamonicapress.com

Printed in the United States

Santa Monica Press books are available at special quantity discounts
when purchased in bulk by corporations, organizations, or groups.
Please call our Special Sales department at 1-800-784-9553.

This book and its website are intended to provide general information. The
publisher, author, distributor, and copyright owner are not engaged in rendering
health, medical, legal, financial, or other professional advice or services. The
publisher, author, distributor, and copyright owner are not liable or responsible to
any person or group with respect to any loss, illness, or injury caused or alleged to
be caused by the information found in this book and its website.

ISBN-13 978-1-59580-051-0

Library of Congress Cataloging-in-Publication Data

Lewis, Simon (Simon R.)
Rise and shine : the extraordinary story of one man's journey from near death to
full recovery / Simon Lewis. — 2nd ed.
    p. cm.
Includes index.
ISBN 978-1-59580-051-0
1. Lewis, Simon (Simon R.)—Health. 2. Brain damage—Patients—United
States—Rehabilitation. 3. Brain damage—Patients—United States—Biography.
4. Television producers and directors—United States—Biography. I. Title.
RC387.5.L49 2010
617.4'81044092—dc22
[B]

                              2009043165

Cover and interior design and production by Future Studio

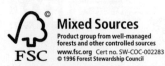

Mixed Sources

Product group from well-managed
forests and other controlled sources
www.fsc.org Cert no. SW-COC-002283
© 1996 Forest Stewardship Council

RISE AND SHINE

The Extraordinary Story of One Man's Journey from Near Death to Full Recovery

Simon Lewis

CONTENTS

INTRODUCTION 7

CHAPTER ONE: MEET JOHN DOE........................... 13

CHAPTER TWO: INNERSPACE................................ 33

CHAPTER THREE: BY DAWN'S EARLY LIGHT..................... 47

CHAPTER FOUR: THE BUSINESS OF CARING................... 51

CHAPTER FIVE: IN MY ROOM 57

CHAPTER SIX: DESPAIR 63

CHAPTER SEVEN: A HIGH-ACUTE PATIENT 67

CHAPTER EIGHT: MEANING.................................. 75

CHAPTER NINE: FEAR, AND HOPE 91

CHAPTER TEN: HOME 101

CHAPTER ELEVEN: FASTER, HARDER, BETTER 109

CHAPTER TWELVE: MEET DOCTOR FEELGOOD 129

CHAPTER THIRTEEN: FALSE PROPHETS 163

CHAPTER FOURTEEN: WESTERN AND EASTERN RECOVERY 177

CHAPTER FIFTEEN: **HARRISON FORD**............................ 191

CHAPTER SIXTEEN: **TURNING POINT** 199

CHAPTER SEVENTEEN: **DEUS EX MACHINA** 215

CHAPTER EIGHTEEN: **WHEN TWO AND TWO MAKE FIVE**..........237

CHAPTER NINETEEN: **AN OPEN MIND**............................. 261

CHAPTER TWENTY: **WHERE TECHNOLOGY AND LIFE UNITE**.......283

CHAPTER TWENTY-ONE: **FULL RECOVERY: MIND, BODY, AND SOUL** 307

CHAPTER TWENTY-TWO: **CONFLUENCE** 321

ACKNOWLEDGMENTS 329

DISCLAIMER................................ 331

GLOSSARY 333

RESOURCES..................................347

FICTIONALIZED NAMES 349

INDEX 351

For everyone who needs to find the hidden path

INTRODUCTION

When I was thirty-five, my wife and I were both reported dead by the first paramedics to arrive at the scene of a seventy-five-mile-an-hour hit-and-run. My wife Marcy died instantly that day. With brain damage from a massive stroke and my body broken, I wasn't expected to survive either. As a producer, I developed films all the way from a blank page to completed movie, but that night it was my parents, with a son in intensive care, who confronted the blankest page imaginable.

The journey began in a strange, unfamiliar place. My stroke, brain surgery, and month-long coma damaged my memory and my reason, the senses that define who I am. Before this, my memories were like precious photos, arranged in sequence through my life; now the album in my mind felt empty, almost every photo shaken out into a jumble of amnesia. I was a visitor from another planet, an observer of life unable to participate in it. Some describe such victims of brain injury as "walkie-talkies," except I was bedridden, too.

Before I understood why, I tried to find my lost memories; I made notes on scraps of paper late at night when subconscious thoughts surfaced, especially after major surgeries, when deep anesthesia took me on repeated trips—as many as fifteen times—down, and then back up, the slope of consciousness.

Piece by piece, fragments from the innerscape of my coma returned with me from each trip and took shape; in time, the scraps of paper multiplied. I have them still, scribbled memos of my mind that I arranged on my parents' dinner table when I began this book. Maybe the search for memories kept me sane, helped me face Marcy's death and the loss of almost everything that made my life precious. For as I explored treatment options to rebuild my future, I found few answers.

"No head injury is too severe to despair of, nor too trivial to ignore," said Hippocrates, the founder of medicine way back in the 4th century BC, though few doctors share this ancient wisdom with patients today. When actress Natasha Richardson shrugged off hospital tests after she fell on a gentle bunny ski-slope, it was a commonly missed intervention for a condition doctors call "talk and die," because the patient declines so fast.

Stephen, a healthy man I knew, tripped over his cat in the dark one night and cut his forehead. After the emergency room sent him home he lived with no sign of illness—and no diagnosis—for sixteen weeks; then mentioned in his diary some "double vision," and a need for new glasses. Soon after, with no prior history of strokes, he died of one in his sleep.

Another acquaintance of mine described a single knock on his head from the handle of his tree pruner; how he blacked out for a moment and went back to pruning his backyard with a bruise on his temple as the only visible change, until this "trivial" injury triggered partial brain seizures that changed his life. These three cases illustrate the extent of uncertainty Hippocrates described, and about which we know little more today.

For as I emerged from my stroke and coma, I met specialists who practiced only their specialty, and from within it issued reports that measured me, but didn't describe what was wrong, or how to fix it. Something as basic as the extent of my injuries, or the cause of my headaches, might not be known for years, and they gave no vision of my potential, or life ahead. I didn't know how much my mind and body could heal, how long it might take, or how to influence where my path to recovery would end. I discovered that America pays the least of all developed nations for rehabilitation care and, as overstretched providers offered a kaleidoscope of opinions, I learned how little physicians understand the path to full recovery, one that might allow my body and brain to repair.

Yet dissect a nerve on a jellyfish, and it will heal just like a paper cut on your finger; it will even regrow a perfect new jellyfish body part. So I wanted to understand the ultimate limits on my recovery. Why, if I was able to grow my brain once, I shouldn't be able to grow it again. And if my brain was this powerful self-organizing tool—I hoped a bit more advanced than a jellyfish—could it overcome my stroke to recover the skills I needed?

The answers lie inside our genome, the tiny universe inside each of us. All the DNA in your body unraveled would reach from the Earth to the Sun and back many times over, but no one knows the momentary cascades, the hidden protein paths in our cells that make life possible. Doctors are still at the dawn of understanding how far each of us can heal. The extent of my recovery, that began the night I was crushed between a truck and a tree, was hailed as a miracle, but it also flowed from medicine. I've respected the privacy of some treatment providers who asked me to fictionalize their names, and otherwise wrote this book with the information I used to achieve my recovery, in order to share the knowledge that I wish someone had given me. For as weeks turned to months, and then to years, I learned by trial and error to ask some of the right questions about my migraines and fears; to weigh medical opinions that often conflicted; to understand how medical insurance really works, and secure coverage for treatments with the best outcome. So this is both the story of my full recovery, and what I learned as I searched for the hidden path to it.

I hope this book helps you or someone you love find that path. It is well hidden. From the first paramedic who raced to our car, I could not have imagined the doctors and therapists I would discover, some in specialties I didn't know existed, nor the breakthrough technologies they used to help me heal, many not widely known or adopted.

At times I feared I was on a delusional search for El Dorado; that, in fact, there was no chance of full recovery, no spiritual city of gold. And at those moments of crisis I was totally grateful for my family, for without their encouragement and love I could never have achieved success. In 1994, an unknown world lay ahead, and their unwavering support empowered me never to give up, but to go forward, explore the issues, and find that hidden path.

While I've edited some events, I've tried to write an honest book. Not all victims recover. I miss Marcy every day and this book is dedicated to her memory, to the special light she brought into my life, in the hope it may help other survivors, at all levels of injury, find their way forward to tomorrow. During a search that took me to people and places I never dreamed existed, the notion of a path to full recovery of my mind and body grew from wishful hope to certainty. As I followed it, I learned a beautiful truth: If you treasure your life, finding how to enjoy good physical and mental health, every day, is the ultimate treasure hunt.

No matter how hard the road you travel, wherever your journey takes you, I wish you and those you love all the health to be unlocked from your genome, when you find the hidden path.

CHAPTER ONE

MEET JOHN DOE

"They're funny things, accidents," said Eeyore.
"You never have them 'til you're having them."
—A.A. Milne,
The House at Pooh Corner

"Like me to show you the Music Center president's new home?" Marcy asked with her bright laugh.

We had met a year and a half before, separately invited to a weekend party at Lake Tahoe, and Marcy was my passenger. When our car reached Magic Mountain on the return trip, I asked her for a date, and after a happy courtship, proposed in her hometown of Phoenix. Married for five brilliant months, tonight was to celebrate our first new car, which we picked up two days before from the Infiniti dealer. My bride was the marketing director for the Music Center, the Performing Arts Center of Los Angeles County, and her boss's new home nearby was an architectural sight.

"Let's take a look after dinner," I suggested, hungry after a day in class with USC's graduate film students.

We were headed west on Beverly Boulevard, a major six-lane road that crosses L.A., a few blocks from Farfalle, the restaurant where I threw Marcy a surprise birthday party. Her friends serenaded her from the balcony above the back dining patio, and it was our favorite since.

You never get to make the two decisions of real importance in your life: how you arrived, and when you will leave. We always die too soon or too late, our life complete at that moment. And in that moment, Marcy left. A disabling or fatal injury strikes someone in America every two seconds. On film and television, death usually involves suspense. Some appropriate dialogue, a ticking clock, or an assassin in the shadows as music and editing slowly build to climax. But in real life, there's no foreshadowing, no hint of what's to come. We live our lives in that single moment in which the present becomes our past, perhaps why we call it "the present," for there are infinite possibilities within every moment it gives us.

If I paused to tighten my shoelaces before I left USC to collect my wife from work, we would have been twenty feet back and missed the speeding bullet headed toward us. *If* we caught one more red light on our route, we would have reached our restaurant safely. But in that moment, on that day, I was behind the wheel of a brand new four-door Infiniti, as we drove along a typically busy thoroughfare, those few short blocks from Farfalle.

It was just before 7:00 PM. That moment, a young couple was about to cross McCadden Place, a quiet residential side street running north-south lined with trees that feeds into Beverly Boulevard. Shaded by the maples, it's the sort of leafy two-lane road that's safe for kids to play on, with homes down both sides and stop signs at either end; the kind of street you can step into when you cross at the same time as you check for traffic. Except right then, an unregistered white Chevy van hurtled north on it at seventy-five miles an hour, gas pedal floored. It blew through the stop sign and sliced through the first four of Beverly's six lanes. But for our Infiniti that blocked the Chevy's path, it would have crossed the last two lanes—the final thirty feet of Beverly—and taken the young couple. Instead, it broadsided us, the worst kind of collision.

The sound of the crash froze the young couple's steps, and they watched the truck smash the Infiniti onto the far side of Beverly Boulevard, bulldozing it across the final two lanes. The force was immense. When the Infiniti's wheels ground against the curb, the Chevy still powered forward, and the pinned Infiniti had nowhere to go except up. So when it reached the curb, the Infiniti took off and, airborne, arced twenty feet until it smashed into the big maple in front of the house at the corner. The rigid tree delivered a second crushing body blow to the other side of our car, completed the last coincidence, and final *if*.

There was no pain for me as death began. The brain doesn't feel pain in that way, but swells when traumatized. And the more damage it suffers, the more ruptured blood vessels leak, the more oxygen the brain needs, and the more it swells. Encased within the skull, it can't expand, so increasing pressure damages, then destroys, more brain tissue. And because of its position in the skull, the pressure tends to push the brain down into the opening that connects with the brain stem, then jam the brain stem in turn through the base of the skull, into the spinal canal.

The Bergen family had started dinner in the

house at the corner of Beverly and McCadden when they felt the explosive concussion. As soon as the ground shook, they ducked under their table for cover from, they thought, an earthquake, except the tremor ended too fast. They looked out their window, and saw the Infiniti where it landed in front of their home.

Harvey and Joy Warren, married film writers, were also on their way to dinner.

As their manager and producer when I represented writers and directors at Blake Edwards Entertainment, I'd set up some deals for them and we'd become good friends. Harvey saw a white van apparently parked normally by the side of Beverly, and then did a double take.

It was like one of those kid puzzles, "What's wrong with this picture?" From where he sat, the Chevy looked quite normal—except its spinning wheels weren't on the road, but at the top. This Chevy was parked on its roof. Once Harvey drove past it, saw the wreckage and understood, he pulled over, grabbed his fire extinguisher, and raced like a good Samaritan toward a river of gas that gushed from the back of the Infiniti.

The car's frame had imploded, and crushed me into an impossibly small space between the driver door and center console, chest and face jammed into the steering column, my airbag deployed and bloody. There was no sound, no movement, so they turned to Marcy. A letter Joy wrote to my parents described what she and Harvey saw that I will never remember, and can never change:

> *An off-duty paramedic came onto the scene, discovered the passenger was not breathing and immediately began CPR through a plastic mouthpiece. People came running out, thinking there had been an earth-*

quake. The paramedic screamed for some-one to call 911.

A young woman in her car said she had 911 on her car phone. She screamed, 'Don't move anyone, under any circum-stance.' But the passenger wasn't breath-ing. The paramedic said he had no choice but to move her enough to administer CPR to try and revive her.

Neither the passenger nor the driver could have been moved without taking the car apart anyway. Harvey knew that the passenger, Simon's wife, wasn't going to survive—despite the seat belts, despite the airbags. It was a terrifying sight in a resi-dential neighborhood.

A parking control officer who hap-pened to be writing tickets in the neighbor-hood arrived on the scene. I handed him some flares from our trunk, to set up traffic control. And we waited some more.

Finally a fire truck arrived on the scene. Still no ambulance or police. The firemen counseled against the flares, even out in the street, and said they would take over now.

Had we known it was Simon—and, God help him, Harvey was not even two feet from him and couldn't tell it was him—we would have stayed on and tried to make sure every effort was made in his and Mar-cy's behalf. We thought we were just in the firemen's way at this point.

Another observation. We were there fifteen to twenty minutes. When we left, the police still had not arrived. . . .

The paramedic was on his way to work at Cedars-Sinai Medical Center less than a mile away, and witnessed the crash. He couldn't reach me when he raced to our car, and so he focused on Marcy, who in a cruel irony appeared peacefully asleep as he unsuccessfully attempted CPR.

"Two vehicles. No survivors," he sighed as her life slipped away. With no survivors, there was no reason for 911 to dispatch an ambulance, and no hope for my remains, buried motionless and silent deep inside the mangled car, as the firemen waited for the siren of their salvage truck. California leads the nation in hit-and-runs, and L.A. leads the state by far.

Of the two million Americans who suffer traumatic brain injury (TBI) each year, most from car and motorcycle accidents, up to a hundred thousand will die prematurely. Many will face up to a decade of extensive rehabilitation, often to restore only minimal function, because even a TBI as seemingly minor as a concussion can have devastating long-term physical, as well as mental, consequences.

To the rescue team that arrived, I looked far beyond the point of no return. With two Jaws of Life systems, it would take more than another hour for them to spread open and cut apart the twisted scraps of what was once our car. While they worked, police investigated the brand new Infiniti with untraceable dealer plates; no access to the lifeless driver for license or other identification, and the Owner's Manual in the glove box not yet completed. "UNK," they wrote in most of the boxes on their Traffic Collision Report. "Unknown," like the main character's name in Kurt Vonnegut's *Sirens of Titan*, a book I had discussed adapting into a movie after my current project *Mother Night*. As for the missing Chevy driver, he bought the white van days before at a car lot. Through a gap in the registration system favored by dealerships, there was no obligation for them to verify a car buyer's identity or insurance. So this guy paid cash, drove the Chevy straight off the lot, killed my wife, and escaped into the night.

There would be legislation, helped into law by my father and others' testimonies before the California Senate in Sacramento, to allow police to impound such vehicles and take dangerous drivers off the road, but too late for us. We were now a file with sixty police photos; the Personal Effects Inventory of what was in our pockets; and a death certificate as Marcy was taken from my side on her final path: "DOB 07/27/1966, died 03/02/1994, Multiple Blunt Force Body Trauma."

Intermittent traffic flow was restored as rescue crews cleared debris. Dr. Phil Anderson of Cedars-Sinai, on his way to work like the first paramedic, looked out his car window and wondered if he'd get a call on this one.

When the Jaws of Life crew cut off the driver's door, and a first rescuer reached in his fingers to touch my cold nonresponsive wrist, he felt a faint pulse. I was still alive, still dying, my body temperature in deep hypothermia. Amid all the unknowns, I believe lack of access helped save me; the fact paramedics couldn't physically get to my body and wrap it in blankets to try to keep me warm, to stop the process of my death, let my brain and body shut down.

One element of the medical protocol, applied as soon as the team got to me, may also have saved me. In America, the protocol is to evacuate victims in critical condition—even at the risk of immediate death as paramedics lift their broken bodies onto stretchers—because getting them to full medical facilities is their best chance. I'll always be grateful for the do-or-die, proactive American approach.

For now, the extraction team sheared off the roof

and all doors, cut through the seat belt and my clothes to reach my body. All belongings left behind in the car's stripped hull, I was naked and nameless, balanced between death and rebirth, as the ambulance team tried to maintain key functions, keep me breathing with a tightly sealed bag-valve mask and flow meter to force feed pure oxygen. Cedars-Sinai was close—less than a mile—but after three hours, blood began to trickle from my ears as the pressure inside my head passed critical.

The largest nonprofit hospital in the western United States, Cedars-Sinai spans several city blocks. Despite all the medical cutbacks, it was one of the few remaining fully equipped trauma center ERs and, because it wasn't the weekend, it had room for me. Two more life-saving factors added to the balance, in which my fate now lay.

"Moving all extremities and phonating unintelligibly, but not verbalizing," the admission report read. Straight into the Intensive Care Unit they raced me, to waiting doctors and critical care nurses—the full resources of modern American medicine in a great hospital, poised to deploy at full speed.

On the wall of every ICU is a big clock. All is done to the clock, including the time of death, but until that point the team methodically goes through its steps; doctors make choices, ICU nurses are trained to never say so much as "oops!" always "there!" if they drop something. All highly trained soldiers of life, they were ready to take control of my breathing and blood circulation with full intubation, but they had no identification, no medical history, and no assessment of my internal injuries. Fatal seizures after brain injury are common, and inevitably there were two schools of thought: Whether to use anti-seizure drugs immediately, which may increase the risk of later seizures, or to wait until they happen.

My doctor chose to follow the second theory, perhaps because any further disruption to my brain chemistry looked too risky. Once they met my critical needs, they could attempt to sedate me, try to move me onto life support, and only then could they prepare me for the next level of care.

The development of films and television shows is often a family business. To keep costs down through the time between movies, while I developed and wrote fresh projects and lectured at USC, my mother would field calls and maintain the offices. She'd worked years before in the British film business, and it was light work she enjoyed.

At the end of that day, as I drove off the USC campus to collect Marcy, my mother confirmed to film director and star Keith Gordon and his producer Bob Weide that I'd set a meeting on *Mother Night* with Sony Classics first thing next morning. She'd called Marcy and me twice at our home and gone to bed, wondering why I hadn't called in to confirm I'd be there. It was after 11:00 PM when the phone rang, and she heard the harsh static of a two-way radio car phone.

"Who's there?" my mother asked.

"Is this . . . Mrs. Patricia Lewis?" a voice answered.

"Yes, who are you?"

"Are you alone?" the voice pressed.

"No, I'm with my husband. . . . Who is this?" my mother insisted, confused.

Pause, more static.

"May I speak to . . . Mr. Basil Lewis?" the voice persisted.

"Not until you tell me who you are."

There was a longer pause, then a new voice on the line.

"This is Detective Pearson, West Traffic Division. . . . Marcy Lewis is dead and your son is critical."

My mother broke down. My father took the phone from her and confirmed the facts. He belongs to what Tom Brokaw called The Greatest Generation in his book about everyday people who were transformed by the challenges of World War II, as in my father's case when he was plucked from the London School of Economics to serve in the British Army in Burma. The double tragedy was overwhelming for them, as it is for the millions who get an unexpected call from the police. My father took my mother's hands.

"Our son is still alive, and he needs us to be strong for him," he said gently.

A great man in every sense, he already knew his next urgent step. My parents were in Sherman Oaks, at least a half-hour from Cedars. Between their two other sons—my brother David, an attorney, and Jonathan, a financial consultant—David in Beverly Hills was nearest to the hospital.

Within seconds, David had the information and called his next-door neighbor, Mark Neame, a doctor who practiced there. Dr. Neame was a gastroenterologist I'd met at my brother and sister-in-law's home.

"Mouth to anus, liver to pancreas!" he'd humorously introduced himself. Like an Elizabethan courtier making a formal bow, his hand marked out in the air the north, south, east, and west of the digestive system with a flourish as he described his medical specialty. When Mark's wife answered the phone, David spoke calmly, clearly.

"Ruth, it's David. Medical emergency. I need Mark."

And seconds later, "Mark, my brother is in critical condition at Cedars."

Mark expected more details, and questions, but then realized David was done. That was all the information that mattered. Mark cut to the bottom line.

"Be at your front door in five, ready to leave."

When Mark arrived, he took David into a room away from the kids, then called Cedars, gave his medical code, and connected to Intensive Care.

"Who's on duty? Good. I need status on Simon Lewis."

"No Simon Lewis here tonight," countered the duty nurse, as she checked her register.

Mark frowned, and picked up the handset to disable the speakerphone. "Run your John Does," he said quietly.

Different ages, sexes, and ethnicities flowed inaudibly down the phone line; a roll call of those touched by catastrophe that day.

"Next, next," Mark intoned, until he heard about a male Caucasian, John Doe #584291, date of birth 00/00/0000, estimated in his thirties.

He hung up, turned to David, and chose his words. "Some good news. We have the 'A Team' in the ER tonight. Let's go."

After a quick call to my parents, the two headed for Cedars. While David drove, Mark worked the cell phone, got more data on this John Doe, and based on it, began to track down a colleague who might save my life. Assuming you're an average adult, if you laid out all your blood vessels in one line, they would be close to a hundred thousand miles long, driven by your heart, beating more than a hundred thousand times a day. Interventional radiologists are medical detectives, specialists in imaging trauma victims, who try in a desperately short time to find the critical breaches in that hundred thousand mile, three-dimensional latticework, and embolize, or seal, them.

Of over a thousand doctors who practiced at Cedars, there were only a couple of interventional radiologists, and Mark reached Dr. Richard Van Allan at his home to come out in the middle of the night to this John Doe.

As he listened to Mark, and urged his Jaguar through the streets of Beverly Hills as fast as he could, David felt encouraged. He heard the "A Team" had successfully transferred me onto full life support, and assumed my life was saved with Mark's interventional radiologist on his way into the ICU "stat"—the highest medical priority. Mark decided to adjust David's expectations, and reveal the side of his conversations that my brother didn't hear.

"David, your brother's blood loss is massive, and it hasn't stopped," he explained. "The surgeon says that as fast as his transfusions inject new blood, it leaks out again through Simon's internal injuries."

As they pulled into Emergency Admissions, Mark described how a patient whose blood pressure dropped this low went into irreversible shock. Even with transfusions, a patient who loses too much blood reaches a point of no return, and their life ebbs away.

In the ICU, the team managed to control John Doe enough to run critical care images of his head, jaw, chest, ribs, pelvis, knees, and feet. His whole body was crushed, every cavity filled with blood. A hematoma is the collection of blood in tissues or space following the rupture of a blood vessel. In the brain, they can be epidural (or outside the brain and its fibrous covering, which is called the dura); subdural (between the brain and its dura); or intracerebral (in the brain tissue itself).

The scans revealed John Doe had all three, generalized brain swelling with massive, diffuse injury to it. Perhaps a third of the right hemisphere was already destroyed, containing his parietal lobe, where we process multi-sensory input to create an integrated picture of our environment so we feel embodied within it; and close by the frontal lobe, involved in planning, problem solving, personality, and a variety of higher cognitive functions, including behavior and emotions.

All were damaged to an unknown extent in this John Doe as the pressure in his brain built, unrelentingly, for over four hours. Blood pumped into the spaces behind his sockets, giving John Doe what doctors call "raccoon eyes," bulging and black.

Eyes wide open, the irises were asymmetric, empty of apparent thought or personality as his crippled brain began to lose control of its autonomic systems, the patterns acquired by the brain stem at the dawn of consciousness. There was more blood now from his nostrils and ears as the intracranial pressure, or ICP, steadily rose.

The "A Team" neurosurgeon, Dr. Bruce Kern, stood by, scrubbed in and ready to open the skull. But with no medical history available, he needed to wait for clearance to go in. He had to know if it would kill the patient. More specialists arrived in the Intensive Care Unit, from Dr. Kern down to Dr. Ramsay, the resident on duty that night, as Cedars is also a teaching hospital. With a gross incision opened through the abdominal cavity, the general surgeon confirmed the status of John Doe's major organs.

Liver, spleen, stomach, and kidneys were in place, and apparently functional. A shadow on an image required Kern to wait more, until an emergency aortogram checked John Doe's heart; also still functional. At last, he got the green light for ventriculostomy, a procedure to measure the pressure inside of the skull by placing a device within one of its fluid-filled, hollow chambers and, once measured, to release and then regulate the pressure.

Dr. Van Allan checked his scans, as he gained access to the blood vessels, snaked his guide wire and catheter through arteries, and tried to find the sources of bleeding deep within John Doe's pelvis, as blood spurted and leaked its way through his ruptured circulatory system. The heart forces our blood on its steady journey all our life, but now—*thump, thump, thumpety-thump*—the artificial pump pushed it through John Doe, and out again. With continuous transfusions, this John Doe needed more than forty-five units (more than four replacements of every drop in him), plus multiple packs of plasma. And even after Van Allan's catheter injected an embolizing agent to seal the main leaks and preserve arterial flow, the team would have to wait and see, because it takes hours for banked blood to restore its crucial flow of oxygen to body tissue.

There were eight operating rooms on four different floors at Cedars-Sinai, all deserted as David and Mark ran through them in search of John Doe until they entered this one, and changed into scrubs. My brother was familiar with operating rooms. Long before he became an attorney, he was a summer intern in the operating room of a brain surgery hospital, but was still not prepared for what he saw.

The body was black and blue from head to toe due to internal bleeding and bruises. The lucky number 7 represents the seven openings of the human body, but when you're fully intubated in the ICU, every one of them is managed by machines and sealed—your luck run out. For Ian Fleming, creator of Agent 007, the "00" signified the eyes, hence the classic opening of the Bond movies. John Doe's asymmetric black eyes were now shut. But none of this was what most shocked David: The whole body was double-sized, inflated like some bizarre Stay Puft Marshmallow Man, as though the ventilator had blown John Doe up like a child's balloon.

"Yes," David confirmed, "that's Simon Lewis. . . . That's my brother."

Mark turned to the "A Team" anesthesiologist,

Dr. Alan Sloane.

"Do the best you can for him. He's a friend."

Later that year, when one of his children asked him to talk about his most rewarding work for a school project, Sloane would describe this night; his attempts to stabilize a disfigured John Doe with apparently fatal injuries, who at that moment on his operating room gurney became identified, a person with a family. No longer John Doe #584291, date of birth 00/00/0000, but someone's *friend*.

Dr. Brien, the team's orthopedic surgeon, introduced himself to my brother to get David's consent to treatment. In critical care, treatment often begins before there's anyone to ask, so doctors are sometimes required to get consent for procedures they've already performed. Brien needed David's immediate approval for the decisions that had already been made and implemented.

"Normally I can stop the bleeding by oversewing the arteries," he explained. "But that's impossible. Simon's pelvis is crushed. At this level of trauma, there're two choices to try and save him. I'm supposed to either inject surgical gel into his body—attempt to seal his blood vessels inside—or I can apply compression around the exterior of his body, and try to stop the bleeding from outside."

David saw the man's exhaustion, and heard the gravity that lay in those tentative words, *try and save him*. And wondered which course of action Brien took.

"Get control of the bleeding from inside, or from the outside. One or the other," he repeated carefully. There was a choice to be made, and Dr. Brien wanted the patient's caregiver to both know and approve his decision.

"I didn't think either would be enough to save your brother," he concluded grimly, "so I elected to do both. That's why he's so bloated. His body's filled with pressurized gel—*and* his extremities are pinned with tourniquets."

"What happens next?" David asked, as he looked at my barely recognizable body.

"Now, we have to hope for the best," Brien replied, and turned back to his team.

There are rules that limit what doctors can tell patients, and after they left the ICU, Mark turned to my brother.

"I'm sorry, David," he confided, "but I think you should know. No one in ICU thinks Simon will make it."

Dr. Brien and his team had, Mark explained, listed the multiple procedures they would attempt if I stabilized. That was their strategy, except no one in the room thought I would stabilize, live through the procedures if I did, or that the outcome could be changed. I wasn't expected to survive through the night, let alone be brought back. When my other brother, Jonathan, reached the hospital and hurried into the sterile waiting area, David took him to one side.

"Don't go in, laddie," he said softly. "You don't want to see this . . . see him this way." His voice and expression made clear they could do no more for me, and Jonathan understood. It was the first separation; for my two brothers to remember me as I was, not for what now lay in the ICU, and to prepare to accept that my future would exist only in their memories of me. David told my parents the same when they arrived.

And they all waited as the waiting room gradually emptied, until my parents told David and Jonathan to go home, and then my parents waited more, alone in the hushed stillness as my life hung in the balance.

It was 1:00 AM by the time Kern decided he could attempt his emergency craniotomy to remove the multiple hematomas and secure the bony fragments of my shattered skull with eight tiny plates. It was the most delicate surgical procedure possible, and throughout, he carefully watched the ICP monitor he'd inserted to minimize further brain damage.

Six hours later, scans showed successful evacuation of the hematoma. Kern stepped out of the OR to my mother, who had long since persuaded my father to go home to get some sleep, and waited alone in the early dawn light of the hospital hallway.

"Mrs. Lewis, I think Simon might live, but he will be completely paralyzed—at least down the left side of his body."

"Then pull the plug. End his life support," my mother urged, distraught.

"But I thought he was an attorney? He can still live a productive life."

Kern was tired, confused. It was not the reaction he expected. My mother was clear, desperate.

"He wouldn't want to come back like that—I know my son," she begged. "Please, Doctor. *Let my boy go.*"

She was right. I'm not a brave man. Many brave people live with great difficulty, but that, in all honesty, would not be my wish. I've always believed the truth of Neil Young's lyric: "It's better to burn out than to fade away. . . ."

Easier to be taken off life support, burn up in an instant, happy with the memory of Marcy at my side, than for my paralyzed body to fade away. As Clint Eastwood's Harry Callahan character said in *Magnum Force*, "A man's got to know his limitations," and I know mine. I don't have the guts it takes, and would want the easy way. If all life must end, let mine end here, peacefully, so that my family could move on without me. My mother knew it.

"Please, Doctor, turn off the life support," she

begged.

But in the event, I wasn't asked.

"I'm sorry. It's not my department," Kern replied, and slipped away. Doctors learn how to disappear where patients and caregivers cannot follow—into the "doctors only" areas of the hospital, backstage from the public.

With the star neurosurgeon and his team gone for the night and my condition not yet stable for the next, orthopedic level of surgeries, there now remained in the ICU only Dr. Ramsay. The overworked, under-appreciated resident—a doctor-in-training—is the most junior member of the ICU team, and this was his very first time in charge; mine the first unstable life left en-tirely in his hands. None of his state of the art machines could trace the threads of my consciousness. Modern medicine cannot see inside our minds, and from outside, his patient looked completely inert, lost to the world.

Dr. Ramsay would tell me one day how he began to watch the life support dials, and the ventilator that sighed softly over my bloated body, just like his pro-fessors instructed him in the classroom; then panicked when the reality broke through of his situation. Every-one else had left the room and dropped total responsi-bility for my life onto his shoulders alone. He'd describe how he calmed himself, and made a solemn resolution.

"I hadn't slept since my twenty-hour shift began," he explained, "and I decided I wasn't going to lose my first case. I wouldn't let go of you—no matter what."

He wouldn't sleep, wouldn't allow the vital signs to deviate, then flatline to end my life because he stepped away for more coffee. No, he wouldn't take his eyes off those monitors. He began to make small adjustments to maintain perfect homeostasis, and steeled himself to his long vigil, as my guardian angel.

In accordance with the customs of my religion, I would be renamed Life to commemorate my new birth into the world when I was saved that night, and a prayer inserted into the Wailing Wall in Jerusalem for me. But as Ramsay watched the EEG trace my unstable brain patterns, still in critical condition, and looked at my crushed form with all its tubes as they snaked in and out, he must have had questions.

There could be no answers from the Marshmallow Man in the oxygen mask, only the steady beep of the monitors, but he had to wonder. What was still inside me? Who was I now? Where was I?

CHAPTER TWO

INNERSPACE

Like a circle in a spiral
Like a wheel within a wheel
Never ending or beginning
On an ever-spinning reel
As the images unwind
In the windmills of your mind
—Dusty Springfield,
"Windmills of Your Mind"

My motionless silence gave no sign of life within, as life support mechanically maintained me at the lowest level of human existence. Though it's a language all of us speak fluently from birth with our thoughts, EEG traces remain silent and mysterious symbols of a foreign realm that communicate with no outsider, and offered doctors and nurses no hint of my progress through those interior worlds.

But as to where I was in that realm, and what I

was during that time, the answer is many places, and
many things. There is no pain in a coma, only a voy-
age that I still remember; a constant exploration of unknown places that are familiar, of unknown people who
accept me. It is a place where everybody knows your
name, and you never need to speak it. The ancients understood. When the Egyptians buried their dead in the
pyramids with objects from their lives, or Norsemen
packed theirs onto a boat and set them ablaze to sink
with those memories, I think somehow they felt what is
true about the afterlife. It is the place you take your life
experiences, and build a new life with them, for that is
what I did—bring fragments of the present, and then a
deeper, puzzling past.

> *I am a pilot. Takeoffs and landings from
> a rooftop, the rush of air surges past me
> as my plane pulls up. And I am released,
> free of everything; high in the mountains
> surrounded by blue sky and white snow
> to a great castle in the mountains, where
> monsters live, where we all celebrate. It is
> Valhalla but I don't know it, complete with
> my lifelong memories of what goes on in
> the castle, the breathtaking sights I have
> beheld here, for it is my home, alive in the
> very distant past with rustic people who
> befriend me, take me in. They ask no ques-
> tions, and are there to help me.*
>
> *In a moment of thirst, I see a hotel
> in the desert. My mind completes the pas-
> sage. We're on a road, traveling fast in hot
> pursuit, and stopping for juice is the big
> reward.*
>
> *The desert, the sense of thirst, takes
> me to another place of race memory, a pre-*

historic settlement in Israel where I've lived
for many generations, and there is a great
emergency. I am at home here also, with
the council elders.

Early the next morning, in the world outside my
dreamscape, my parents gathered the family around
the hand-carved mahogany dinner table they'd brought
from their house in Wimbledon, my childhood home.
Perhaps the place most families discuss their plans,
it was around this dinner table years before that my
father asked us one evening whether, to build better
futures, we wanted to emigrate to the United States.
It took years of planning, of living out of suitcases, and
frequent moves from one apartment to the next, to
reach California together, as new citizens of our promised land.

The issue that morning was how to cope financial-
ly with the crisis that confronted my family. In shock,
my parents explained to David and Jonathan that until
my medical insurance policy was found, they and my
brothers faced ruin. All their years of work in America
could be wiped out by medical bills they couldn't begin
to envision. The most urgent question was whether,
to preserve the lives and opportunities they sacrificed
years to build for themselves, they must abandon me.
Whether they should flee to London that day and leave
me at Los Angeles County Hospital, to be cared for by
the state. That I would never want to be a burden on
their future, the certainty of my answer if they could
ask me, made it no easier. Since no one at Cedars knew
if I would ever come off life support, or what higher
brain functions could survive inside my paralyzed mind
and body if I ever awoke, they had no choice but to de-
bate the unthinkable. My mother, torn between caring
for her husband, children, and grandchildren, thought

about her choice during her long vigil over my body at the ICU.

"Basil, I don't know if I can ever leave Simon's side . . . ," she began.

My father loved to travel with my mother, and in fact was never apart from her throughout their forty-two-year marriage. Haggard, too, from lack of sleep, he wondered where this led.

"Or leave L.A.," she continued. "So, if you want to go to London or anywhere, anywhere at all . . . I'll stay here in Los Angeles with Simon . . . and you and the boys do what's best for them and their families."

There was silence around the table.

"Only one thing matters now," my father answered evenly, and looked at my brothers with steel in his eyes.

"There's only one plan, boys," he said. "America is our home. You must go to work and go on with your lives. Whatever happens, your mother and I will look after Simon. We must not let this affect the way we live as a family."

My aunt Joy, on vacation in L.A. with my parents, knew that this was no time for visitors. It was she alone who called for a family emergency seat on the next plane back to London, and as Joy left on her flight and the sun rose, my parents, in their grief, began the calls.

Bob Weide, the producer who brought the *Mother Night* film project to me, was stunned when my mother called from the early morning activity of the hospital's waiting room, where she'd returned to be close to her son. The meeting at Sony Classics should go ahead anyway; the show must always go on.

"The film's all yours," she told him.

The Music Center Marketing Department struggled to cope with Marcy's death only hours after she said good night at the office as usual, but for the last time. They rallied to my parents' side, and issued a press release at the hospital to help find justice. As TV stations arrived one after the next to interview my father, he appealed to the reporters for help to find the driver, and launched the Marcy Fund to raise reward money to take him off the road. In addition, the city of Los Angeles unanimously approved a motion to offer a $15,000 reward for information leading to the arrest of suspects. But there would be no leads to his identity, the man Harvey Warren noticed as he sprinted toward the crash with his extinguisher. In the confusion, he thought the man was running to help like him; realized too late he was fleeing the murder scene.

Joy Warren looked up to see her husband Harvey enter their living room that night of the press conference, his face ashen from the evening news. "That was Simon in the car," he kept repeating.

As the first day in the real world passed, more experiences flowed in my innerspace universe:

A town built on the water during Prohibition. My mind has come to America, but it is not an America I have ever seen before; this land has more people and places and is completely visualized. I am helping to run whiskey; the unbroken narrative filled with fantastic vistas, of chases through waterways, liquid highways, to a race over the waters of Hawaii on a fast boat. Time is critical; there's a man here who seems larger than life, a kind monster, and yet somehow I feel he is . . . hollow.

At my wormhole between two universes, of the physical and the mind, my boat sails on, now in Southeast Asia as it

*navigates the Mekong Delta. I feel the trop-
ical heat, hear jungle sounds; the rain is
pattering down from above, and all around
us. There is food on the boat; also a woman.
I cannot see her, but feel her presence, and
know I will be safe with her, if I can only go
up on deck to be with her.*

For some dreams, there were clues from the outside world: the desert juice, some liquid forced onto
my tongue; my first images of flight and escape from a
mask, which was like a pilot's, as rushing air took me to
those altitudes. So perhaps that was the oxygen mask
in the ambulance, easily explained. But as my coma
deepened and death advanced, it stripped away all arti-
facts of conscious perception, peeled away layers of my
mind to uncover deeper race memories, as far back as
the ancients, who sought with possessions to unite their
dead with the memories of their ancestors.

*It's cold, wintry cold, and I see a zoo with
many animals. It's so cold here, like St. Petersburg, and the animals are dying. I am
traveling with a great opera company. It's a
huge production, so big the props and scen-
ery and sick animals travel by train across
Russia. I feel the cold in the forest, see the
white snow and my breath, recognize and
am accepted by all the members of the
troupe, who I have never met before. We arrive at our destination, a splendid mansion
in the country with countless rooms. Plays
are held in one of them for the great family
and their many children who live here. I'm
arriving at the house now, walking in deep
gentle conversation with my host.*

Inside the house, I see our performance stage in the large room, lit by a multitude of gentle, brilliant candles, thousands of points of light. I'm in the play, ready, but once onstage, find I cannot speak. In the opera, the role I play is of a bull, and I wear an ornate headpiece that controls me. The bull I have become rears and bucks its head. An icy blast suddenly sweeps the room, the candles gutter one by one—the points of light all die.

In 2003, I would see the movie *Russian Ark*, and watch three hundred years of Russian history unfold, as if in a dream, in that film's single eighty-seven-minute shot that travels through the Hermitage Museum, the former Winter Palace of the tsars. And at the film's climax, I would watch fifteen hundred guests waltz the night away, at what was to be the last great royal ball in 1913. At one point, the camera goes up on stage during a lavish theatrical performance in the Winter Palace, onto a stage where there were no electric lights, just candles and oil lamps.

I knew this was St. Petersburg in my innerscape, and still wonder how, as a descendant of a family from Eastern Europe and Russia, my mind found this world to inhabit, to recognize as its own when stripped of all senses and freed from its boundaries. Days and nights followed as I slumbered round the clock, and the ventilator gently breathed in and out—terrible days for coma families who wait.

My parents flew with my brother Jonathan to Phoenix to meet Marcy's family for her funeral. Tova, Marcy's friend for life, her bridesmaid who flew in from a work assignment in Rome for our wedding, flew again through the night from Italy to rejoin Marcy and attend to her last needs on earth the way she would have wanted. My wife was laid to rest with a song by Squeeze, one of her favorite groups. Music, Tova knew, that Marcy would want as her final song.

> *She visualized a world ahead*
> *And planned how it would be*
> *She left behind the strongest love*
> *That lives eternally*
>
> *Her beauty found in grace*
> *Today she lives another life*
> *In some fantastic place*

My parents and Jonathan listened to the eulogies and music, and wondered if they would return soon to place me beside her; if I would emerge from my coma, or stabilize enough to survive the orthopedic surgeries Dr. Brien still waited clearance to attempt. I slept on as they returned to L.A., and visited my living remains each day, unmoving, suspended in my own fantastic place.

The Music Center held a ceremony and laid a plaque to commemorate Marcy's service. To this day, if you visit the dancing waters of the Music Center fountains and look west, she is in the front corner, near the Taper Forum stage she loved. Caring people made donations to the Marcy Fund that more than doubled the City's reward in an attempt to find justice, ultimately returned when it became clear the police had no leads.

In a final act to help others escape the fate of so many hundreds of thousands of Americans every year, my father made his trip to Sacramento to testify before the Senate Transportation Subcommittee there, and help pass California's Safe Streets Act of 1994.

Like all who wait for loved ones, a hard reality

for my parents was that they didn't know which of my belongings, if any, I would ever use again. As my coma continued, they reluctantly put my life into storage, including Marcy's possessions, so that my old life would be there for me, if I woke.

Brain damage increases with every minute a patient remains unconscious, so as more days ticked away it became unclear if I'd ever be mentally or emotionally equipped to make decisions about Marcy's effects, and my parents gave them all to her parents. A friend of my mother's who needed an apartment moved into our home.

After ten days and nights of life support with no change in my consciousness, Dr. Brien got authorization to attempt the next level of care. The call went out for Alan Sloane, the anesthesiologist, and Dr. Phil Anderson. Anderson, who looked out his car window on his way to work ten days before and seen the car wreck, could finally return to the ICU to address my smashed jaw.

He needed to wire it together, lock it in place until it set—perhaps the bull's headpiece in my coma, in which I could not speak. The task complete, he signaled the go-ahead to Brien. But when Dr. Anderson looked back, he saw his patient wasn't ready. In that second, my muscles reflexively wrenched free of his wires. My eyes were blank, my face a demented, crooked grin, impervious to the fact that he anchored those wires into bone. To tear free of them endangered the integrity of my skull. Only on his third attempt was Anderson finally successful. He nodded once more to Brien that, after his ten-day wait, he could now begin to cut.

It seems likely that the candles in St. Petersburg blew out one by one as Brien began the first incision and Dr. Sloane, finally, took me down to a deeper anesthesia and darkness.

It would be a marathon, the longest surgery of my recovery. The orthopedic team painstakingly inserted hardware, metal plates screwed into place, to keep some of my broken bones more or less aligned. The biggest bone in my body, the O-shaped pelvis, was cracked in at least four places both in back and in front. Into the humerus, the biggest bone in the arm and broken in three places, they inserted a titanium pin.

Twelve hours later, the team was done and my heart still beat, my skeleton reinforced with titanium bolts. And I remained alive, still in a coma suspended on life support, until I might regain consciousness. Another week passed in the calm flow of hospital routine. My family celebrated each time a tube was removed, and my brain showed it could maintain another life function without it.

With tight budgets and overwhelming demand, medical providers do their best to maintain an appearance of complete professionalism. The result for patients is lots of very visible high technology, with invisible inefficiency, right behind; like state-of-the-art ambulances that don't necessarily take you to the closest ER.

It makes vigilance essential, for like ambulances, hospitals are run on an agenda unseen by the patient. Insurance review committees approve a time for each injury to heal, which they regularly cut shorter. On their schedule, a week later, my team of doctors ordered I be moved to a hospital room, with private duty nurses (known as PDNs) to care for me round the clock. There are no windows and no daylight in intensive care, so the team ordered a private room with a window. They wanted me to see natural light, witness night and day, and observe whether I could learn to differentiate them.

There is a slope of consciousness in our minds, countless levels of awareness within. You catch a glimpse of it when you look at your nails, just at the time when they need to be cut. Far down the slope of consciousness, our mind is aware even of that. We have a sense of ourselves, our whole human envelope, which joins us at the dawn of our cognition and persists until soon after it will end. According to the approved schedule, it was time to move me into daylight, but I was still too far down that slope to be moved, and I didn't respond.

My family coordinated their visits each day to my room, to create a continuous circle of care around my bed. Because of their visits to my silent body at such regular intervals, they were the first to spot something else, at first subtle, but which fast turned ominous, and to raise the alarm. They brought in our family internist, Dr. Frank Terrill, who paged a blood specialist.

The fever rose ever higher, as urgent lab tests showed my white blood cell count spike. Nobody seemed to know why, but the mystery bug could kill me. Emergency surgery was necessary to trace the source of such a massive infection, except in all of Cedars no operating room was available, and instead my doctors tried to keep me alive with nonstop intravenous antibiotics. My parents confronted every doctor on my team in the search for an operating room while I dropped deeper into coma, now mixed with delirium, as the unknown infection swept my body.

It took days of increasingly urgent pleas, before Cedars could race me back into an OR for surgical exploration of my abdomen, and the emergency removal of my gallbladder that by this point, the surgeon noted, was "completely gangrenous."

It established one piece of the pattern I learned in my search for full recovery; that infection leaked through my body undetected, as blood seeped into every cavity.

Now in coma nearly a month, my innerspace continued as seamless convolutions that never repeated, were always fresh and interesting, always familiar.

If only my family as they looked on had known. If only other families could take comfort, that whether their loved one in coma lives or slips away, there is no pain on the journey of our spirit to innerspace; only places of comfort, and places of interest.

> *I am a teacher at a school, the first stirrings of personal memories to reassert themselves over the deeper race memories that approaching death revealed. The school is in session for as long as I can remember, with staff I know, but have never met before, and schoolrooms I know well, though I have never seen them before. Always familiar, and always interesting.*
>
> *The school has to move to a new location, perhaps a subconscious awareness of change when the nurses move me to a fresh room, for the innerspace turns from school to religious foundation, where I feel sheltered and protected. Gradually, miraculously, my mind begins to sense something it knows as time. Time becomes a river that I watch, flowing from the boundless horizon of the future to the present.*

After so long in coma, my brain struggled to assemble patterns. The later stages of coma don't resemble what movies and soap operas have taught us to expect—a deep sleep from which an actor opens their eyes, smiles and speaks, immediately recognizable as the person they were before.

Return to life in the real world demands reassembly and recovery by the brain of two different and very uncertain elements: reaction and cognition. To regain "consciousness," both must be present. But the hard truth about comas, as my parents discovered, is my doctors didn't know if, or how well, I would recover either, as they monitored my progress according to their Glasgow Coma and Rancho Los Amigos scales.

The Glasgow Coma Scale involves three simple tests: eye opening, verbal responses, and movement. Based on them, doctors give patients a numerical value, and consider them to have "mild" brain injury when they score a high 13 to 15. From 15, the Scale goes all the way down to 3, a coma so deep the patient's brain damage is often fatal. It's an assessment reserved for the most severe cases of brain injury and dysfunction, because a patient can score up to 4 if they so much as open their eyes.

My doctors were very clear about my score. I was at Glasgow Coma Scale 3, unchanged since admission to Cedars a month before. But with the gangrene surgically removed, as the white cell count dropped out of danger, I began to creep up the slope of consciousness.

Dr. Kern checked my progress as I stabilized. In the days that followed, my head began to turn, ever so slightly, on my pillow. He revised his opinion a second time. If my brain could re-task the reflex to hold my neck straight, I might recover the left side of my body, to some unknown extent. My eyelids began to flicker. What would be behind them when I opened my eyes? My family now waited, like so many families every year, for who would return to them from innerspace.

CHAPTER THREE

BY DAWN'S EARLY LIGHT

And God said, "Let there be light."
. . . And there was evening and
there was morning—the first day.
—Genesis 1:3–5

My eyes opened. I looked around without curiosity. I didn't feel reborn. This felt like the first time. My inner voice, the person you talk to when you talk to yourself, wasn't there, and I didn't notice. I was purely an observer; a visitor from another planet recording sights for the first time. That is how I felt, with the awe of a newborn child at everything I saw, still with no doubts or questions—a simple, gentle rapture in being able to perceive all things, and that I was present in this moment of time and space to behold them.

A person in the previously empty room asked, "What is your name?"

I heard the words that came from nowhere, but

didn't answer. I knew my identity, knew it even as I
looked out upon the river of time as it flowed deep from
the future back to me, but not by any name. I was, simply, *me*. How could a person just born into this world
have a name? It didn't seem to matter.

"*What* is your *name*?" the voice insisted.

I was so tired.

"Simon," I murmured.

I didn't feel like my name was Simon, didn't know
why I said so, but it seemed that I remembered who
Simon was, and this seemed to be his body.

"Do you know *where* you are?"

Still there, my inquisitor asked a question that
I was sure had no answer. Was it a trick? I wondered.
There was no way I should know, how I could possibly
know, what this place was. The intruder with unanswerable questions was enough to make me feel very
threatened, even though the questions stopped, the voice
fallen silent. Sleep enfolded me. When consciousness returned, the sense of threat was mixed with paranoia.

My parents entered my room, and I recognized
them: another critical test passed. "There are monsters
in the mountains, but no one must know," I entreated
from the shrouded fringes between coma and consciousness.

"I know. I'll take care of it," my mother instinc-
tively replied, and my father backed her up.

It was the right answer, but I wasn't satisfied. I
wanted to tell them there was something strange *outside*
the window. With deepest urgency, my eyes appealed to
them for an answer. With no idea what I saw there, beyond my obvious distress about the window, my parents
said they'd take care of that, too. My brothers visited
next and were relieved when I recognized them also.
The nurses recorded that I didn't know where I was and
apparently didn't care, and was incontinent and amne-

siac, for I'd lost all short-term memory.

On their way home from the hospital, my father turned to my mother.

"I've just realized something," he said. "Simon doesn't know he was in an accident."

I didn't, any more than I remembered the separation of day from night. I didn't notice that my jaw was wired shut, the oxygen feeder clipped to my nose to nourish my brain, the nurses who every fifteen minutes entered to turn me to prevent bed sores, or the many other tubes—catheter, IV, a whole collection of them.

Close by my hand was a nurse-call button, on a control pad that could adjust everything in the room from lights, to the TV, to the height and angle of my bed. Not that I knew, or understood anything beyond the one button that could summon help. When the pad fell off the edge of my bed, and hung from the bed frame by its cord, inches from my fingers, I could not understand where it was because it was out of my sight; my mind had barely emerged from Coma Level 3. To protect me, my parents put a notice on the door that read, "No visitors allowed. Do not refer to patient's wife." They wanted their son to find his past in his own time. So I lay in my bed, a newborn child who didn't know he spent his thirty-sixth birthday in a coma, who wondered only about something outside the window. I'd tried to talk about it to my parents, fretted about it, but didn't know the word for it.

Light. And shadow. I'll never forget when I saw them there for the first time, for so it seemed. I marveled at the light, so intense and beautiful. I could dimly see buildings through the blinds, but it was the light that disturbed and captivated me: It made the blinds glitter and sparkle, disappear, then shine anew.

The nurse asked me again if I knew where I was. The sunbeams on the blinds were so beautiful I was sure now, from the quality of the light. I recognized it.

"The South of France?" I murmured.

God saw that the light was good.

I was wrong about the South of France, but right to wonder about the light and what lay beyond the blinds, in shadow. My world may have stopped, but not the one outside my window.

CHAPTER FOUR

THE BUSINESS OF CARING

All in all you're just another brick in the wall
—Pink Floyd,
"Another Brick in the Wall Part 2"

I thought I understood insurance pretty well. During my years of producing films and television programs, I'd learned the importance of all kinds of it. Insurance is our final answer, and ultimate protector. Critical to filmmaking, it lies at the heart of American medicine and its patients. I knew what happened to uninsured victims who arrive at a trauma center like Cedars. "Stabilize and move to County," is the quiet instruction.

When I was single, I always checked my coverage with care, and as a married couple consolidating our lives, I canceled my policy weeks before the crash when Marcy added me to hers, a Great-West employee plan with the Music Center. Once Mark Neame identified me, I was not "moved to County," because the Music

Center notified Great-West, and started the business of caring's ticking clock.

An experienced insurance executive explained to my family how Great-West's coverage of me was under their Survivor Health Benefit, with no premium for six months. After those were up, I'd be eligible for COBRA benefits for a monthly premium.

COBRA is the federal law that requires insurers to keep offering coverage to policyholders who have become uninsurable. The COBRA premium is very high, but like most victims with no other insurance, I had no choice. To the extent they could follow the terminology, it appeared to my family that so long as I improved and could afford the COBRA premium, I had great health insurance coverage for up to thirty-six months, and nothing to worry about. There were hints of what lay ahead in the hospital bills: Page after page itemized with incomprehensible codes, as Great-West assigned an "Associate Director of Risk Management" to patient number 002/070853468, the number on my hospital wristband.

Risk management was necessary because it cost more than five thousand dollars each day I was in the ICU, and this private room, my new home, was well over two thousand. And that was only the room rate. All medical care provided in it was extra, including the six PDNs who checked my vital signs and turned me over every fifteen minutes. Their bills began to pile up too, at $25 an hour for each, round the clock.

My hospital stay was reviewed by something called "PHCS," which stood for Private Healthcare Systems, located on an aptly named Winter Street in far off Massachusetts. Their first letter was addressed to Marcy at our home, and when told of her death and my incapacity, they edited the address to, "Marcy Lewis Unit c/o Basil Lewis."

The cold reality of the business of caring began with denial of payment for the PDNs as their bill hit $12,550. They weren't "necessary."

> Great-West
> April 8, 1994
>
> Medical necessity is determined solely by Great-West Life. The fact that a doctor may prescribe, order, recommend, or approve a service or supply does not, in itself, make such service or supply medically necessary.

My parents protested and pleaded, explaining that the hospital recommended private nursing for my "care and safety." The carrier pointed to the Cedars-Sinai Conditions of Admission—the small print no patient ever reads, let alone one admitted in coma. As far as the hospital was concerned, PDNs were none of its responsibility.

My parents appealed. They had no choice. Even denial of a small portion of services represented a huge financial burden and threat to them and me. They started to cope with the secondary trauma of caregivers—insurance company voices on the phone, who make life and death decisions based on limited information, followed by life and death decision letters.

> Great-West to date has paid $322,590.06 in medical bills; however, we have denied $12,550.00 of private duty nursing. I have spoken with the Catastrophic Case Manager, Pauline Rossi. She explained it would be nice for many patients to have private duty nursing, but that it was rarely approved.

As costs continued to accelerate, my parents
found themselves in the hands of a Catastrophic Case
Manager, a registered nurse. It was ostensibly Pauline
Rossi's job to assess what was medically necessary for
my care—except that according to Great-West's letters,
she was in Englewood, Colorado, and my family should
address mail to a PO box in Denver.

Letters arrived at irregular intervals from PHCS,
to advise that it approved my hospital admission for a
fixed number of days, and it wasn't long before a second
struggle began, as the insurance carrier tried to raid
Marcy's other insurance to pay my medical bills.

Marcy was an employee with a good insurance
plan. One might expect that if she was injured in an
accident, the insurance company would pay the bills
with no questions asked up to the limit of coverage, but
instead plans typically agree to pay them only if the
employee signs a subrogation agreement, under which
the employer's health plan can take all of the money
an employee recovers from any insurance settlement,
to pay medical bills.

This came to light when a certified letter arrived
from Great-West's Recovery Unit asserting "a first lien
Right of Recovery to any sums paid in settlement or
judgment on your behalf as a result of the accident."
Bottom line: Great-West began to go after any recovery it could find to pay the bills. And since all insurance companies share their data—your lifetime claims
history and mine—via CLUE, the Comprehensive Loss
Underwriting Exchange database, nothing is hidden in
their search for money.

The first struggle over the PDNs would drag
on through the summer. Even though I could choke to
death, unable to reach the nurse call button when it
fell off my bed, or call out for help as my jaw was wired
shut, during those months my father faced a kind of

mini-trial on whether the $12,550 for nurses was medi-
cally necessary, and why regular nursing staff couldn't
provide this treatment. There would be multiple letters
by doctors and my father to fight the denial, until a senior Great-West representative finally relented, and
agreed to pay.

The business of caring, almost from the outset,
questioned even tiny bills.

April 1, 1994

> We recently received a claim in the amount
> of $34.86, rendered in conjunction with
> laboratory tests.
>   These tests are automated and inter-
> pretation is done by a machine. Therefore,
> the professional services of a pathologist
> are not considered medically necessary and
> we are unable to cover these expenses.

My parents were nonplussed. If the doctors at Cedars, who saved my life, decided my case was sufficiently complex to justify a pathologist, a human doctor, to
interpret their test results, they didn't understand why,
in the insurer's view, one that cost under forty dollars
wasn't "necessary." Bills would arrive, then second demands from the accounting department at Cedars, "Payment Notice" blazoned across the page in bold red letters.
The balance allegedly due on one, and the check Cedars
demanded my family remit *immediately* in the enclosed
envelope, was for precisely $26,846.49. Accurate to the
penny, except when my parents urgently challenged it,
Great-West said they already paid Cedars.

In the future, we'd receive many such demand
letters months or even years after the date of service
and my parents would learn how to deal effectively with

carriers, and get insurance for the medical services I needed and was entitled to. One day, I'd learn for myself the real health risks of insurance company insistence on interpretations "done by a machine." I'd learn that for full recovery it makes a critical difference who reads a test and writes the report, because the variance between a human expert's interpretation and a boilerplate automated report can mark the difference between success and failure in the search for the hidden path.

I'd learn how insurance confronts all patients who need long-term treatment with a question each year—whether the carrier will provide or deny a policy renewal—the answer to which is a matter of life and death access to continued healthcare.

At times I'd feel, in part because of the Byzantine complexity of the business of caring, that no one was really in control; it was a freight train that hurtled down the tracks with no engineer in the front car. In back, riding in the caboose, were the doctors, overloaded, paid ever later, and often underpaid at that.

And this was one of the finest insurance carriers in the country, which operated to the highest standards. For Great-West would prove to be well named.

How to survive the business of caring's annual policy renewal, and maintain access to the doctors I needed, would be critical throughout my recovery. All I had in March of 1994 was my arrival in a room with one window, my new home, to begin it.

CHAPTER FIVE

IN MY ROOM

The walls are white and in the night
The room is lit by electric light

—Yaz,
"In My Room"

I knew none of the business of caring's maneuvers outside my window that already threatened my saviors, the PDNs. A man swept into my room, flamboyant and dark-haired to introduce them, a prince followed by his retinue. "Roy . . . and the Saratoga Agency!" he grandly announced, and introduced the seven round-the-clock nurses who now protected my world.

Tamara was one who would take a special interest in me when night came, and help me through those long hours when the hospital fell silent, plus three regular Cedars day nurses, Marka, Melissa, and Karin, all specialists in rehab. As coma dreams moved toward reality, Room 7123 became my home, in the high-level rehab wing of Cedars.

My grandmother used to complain of loneliness and boredom, of how all she had were the four walls, and my brothers and I, with the cruel innocence of youth, joked that she never mentioned the ceiling or floor. But I wasn't bored or lonely because I couldn't achieve either state of mind any more than a goldfish in its bowl. I understood my identity, recognized my parents and brothers, and that was the whole sum of my thoughts.

Marka and Melissa were my primary day nurses ("M & M," I repeated over and over to try and remember their names, without knowing why the phrase seemed familiar). Marka, experienced and spirited; Melissa, a young California blonde; and Karin, a kind and very supportive Asian American, completed my all-American team of ten, not counting the doctors.

My first memory of Marka after that introduction was a question.

"May I give you a bed bath, hon?"

I smiled at her by way of response—my wired jaw made any other answer impossible—without understanding. I thought Marka asked if I wanted a *bird* bath. I wondered why she thought I was a bird, but it seemed to make sense because the process involved almost no water, like how a bird uses dust to clean its wings.

There's a children's story about a giant. His head is in the clouds, his feet locked in the ground, and that was how I felt. My brain injury made one half feel heaven was within me while, far below, my other half was silent. Half of me overwhelmed by the beauty of life and the present, by the wonder of that light as it streamed through my window, while within the silence that shrouded the other half of my mind, memory had lapsed into amnesia, information lost all meaning. Without knowing it, I was stranded in the present, anchored to my bed, unaware even of that.

When Karin finally told me I was in a hospital, I neither knew nor could comprehend how it mattered where I was. It didn't occur to me to wonder why, or notice I couldn't move, not even open my mouth. This room and bed were all I knew.

After some days, I remembered the object on the wall of this hospital room was a clock, that it was used to tell the time, and that Simon Lewis once used it to read the time. I also knew that the person I was now couldn't read the clock. But I felt no concern, still a visitor from another galaxy, because I also felt no sense of time, or how it worked. It still ran, constant and steady, from the distant future to me, here in the present.

Like the song says, "Time keeps on slipping, slipping, slipping, into the future. . . ."

My waking cycles began to extend. I watched night follow day, then turn once more to day. My brain saw a pattern it knew, and far down the slope of consciousness, there was recognition. In the next sleep cycle, my mind shifted as it sensed convulsions in the unbroken river of time, the future that flowed so dependably toward me: it was gone.

I felt terribly alone, that in the still, inky blackness all around me, the river I could no longer see flowed uphill, and a sense, this too could not endure. The waters could not flow up to me, but must always wash past me, then flow on down, lost forever, in a place where they would never touch me again.

In my next waking cycle, I understood the direction of time, as it flows from our present, away from us into our past, from which nothing returns.

There were the lyrics to a Yaz song Keith Gordon and I had licensed for our movie *The Chocolate War,*

*The doors are shut and all the windows
    lock*

The only sound is from the clock
I sit and wait alone in my room

But I didn't know that any more. Or understand what a film was. I had no concept of what a month was, how long one took to pass. My memories did not go back that far. My mother visited daily and understood. The doctors told her it might help to talk about things from my past.

"Would you like to watch the Oscars?" she tried.

I felt only inner confusion.

"What's that?" I mumbled.

She switched track, asked me about my film *Look Who's Talking*, a blank look my only response. The gentlest way to encourage my mind, my parents thought, was to expose me to stories from books I'd read as a child that might trigger recognition; so they brought in movies for me to watch on the player in my room.

It made sense because I didn't remember the real world, and was ready only for the whimsical cartoons and fantasy landscapes of *The Wind in the Willows, The Lion, the Witch, & the Wardrobe*. When our genome is understood perhaps we'll find the foundation of our curiosity, the one that survived in me. I responded to Walt Disney's characters, was curious about Toad of Toad Hall and his friends, and most of all, enjoyed the land of Narnia with its lion. It was a natural and real place to me, not a fantasy. I'd only recently inhabited the body of a bull. The "No Visitors" sign on the door let me live childhood memories for what felt like the first time.

M & M bustled in and out, cheerfully checked vital signs, changed my sheets, and talked about the weather—but never the past. It crept in gently at first, whispering glimpses and little details. From childhood forward, some fragments began to link; that I was from England flowed from recognition of my parents and brothers.

"Wayne Rogers sends you best wishes," Jonathan gently tested me one day.

On Jonathan's introduction, I'd executive produced *Age Old Friends* with the star of *M*A*S*H*. And I reacted to Jonathan's words; recognized Wayne's name from a show five years before, as my mind drew closer to the present. There was still no capacity for thought, no dreams at night when I slept.

But now as I lay awake in bed at night, there was an airport. Not an image, only a sense that I was in one. It wasn't threatening. It didn't make me feel fear or paranoia.

Nothing special occurred to me about this airport; there was no apparent reason my brain repeatedly brought me to this uneventful place. I felt it must be important, but had not the slightest inkling of when or where this experience might have occurred. Other than when I soared into the skies of my comascape, I had no memory I ever flew, even less why an airport concourse meant anything.

I'd give up, my mind would wander to random thoughts, then drift back unbidden to the invisible airport. I could not escape. Whether I looked out my window, or at the Disney cartoon as it ran on TV for the umpteenth time in constant play mode, the sense resurfaced. I didn't understand why my mind so often returned here.

Images finally joined the sense memory. Now the airport of my mind was always full of travelers. I saw a concourse, busy with them. But with an image of this airport came a thought of something overlooked, something important there: something *else*.

I lay for hours in my room on that one question. A comascape resurfaced, a race memory from a far ago time—that I was on a boat, which the currents gently rocked as it explored a dark river and rain poured from above, pattered endlessly on the cabin's roof. The sense returned of a woman protector who was with me on the boat, the one I never made it up onto deck to be with. I realized she was with me in the airport. My protector was here, too. She was with me on the river through the jungle, and before that, too, had never left my side. She was one of the travelers in the airport, I understood that now, and she was traveling with me.

I remembered Marcy without insight or question, and with pure joy and a sense of completion. It was in the hours before dawn. Day and night still meant little, because nurses turned me every fifteen minutes round the clock. So Tamara, my tireless PDN, who fed and turned me through the night, was the first nurse I saw. I could hardly wait to tell her the good news.

"I'm married . . . ," I whispered through wired teeth, "to Marcy!"

I was so happy; a man who had found the woman of his dreams.

"That's very nice, Simon," Tamara smiled in encouragement, and when she returned to the nurse's station she quietly called my parents.

That was my last night with the full happiness of Marcy's love. It was my mother who came in the morning to face her bandaged son, strapped to a bed, too damaged mentally even to question why Marcy wasn't there by my side; why no one so much as mentioned her name, as I happily repeated the news that had sustained me since dawn.

"I'm married. To Marcy."

And my mother had come to do the woman's work few men can face; to take her son's happiness away.

"She died, Simon. You were in an accident . . . and Marcy died," she sobbed.

CHAPTER SIX

DESPAIR

*For never was a story of more woe
Than this of Juliet and her Romeo.*
　　　　　　—William Shakespeare,
　　　　Romeo and Juliet, act 5, scene 3

So many moments of our lives are beyond expression, but like everything else, there's an industry of grief experts armed with terminology that talk about "closure" and cleanly defined "stages of grief." They repeat the cliché that "time heals." Many people, I'm sure, find comfort in counselors, but I didn't feel my grief was something I could define, work through on some kind of schedule, and then move on. I still regard the word "closure" as politically correct fiction, an expectation imposed on people who have suffered by those who have not.

My mind and body were already shattered, and now the joy I felt for only a few hours was crushed. The feeling of loss was beyond any expression that my childlike mind could either form, or understand. There was blank emptiness. Most stories of recovery begin with a patient initially paralyzed by fear, who subsequently takes charge of a battle against their disease, finally to triumph over despair.

In most cases, they have insight regarding their impairment and use this to influence their outside world. But I had neither, and was overwhelmed by the realization I had no control of my destiny, and was powerless to save the woman I loved. So I wept, uncomprehending, desolate tears. My brother David visited.

"Where would you like to go one day?" he asked. "We can have a nice trip."

I didn't know. Though I still had use of my words, I'd no understanding of what tomorrow meant, even less how to form goals for it. As I wept, there came the inevitable question of why this happened to Marcy and me, what we did to deserve this. But does anyone ever, at the end of a normal day, look up and wonder why no disaster befell them? And if you don't fill with wonder as the sun sets on all those good days, there's no reason to question the tragic one, the day on which each *if* relentlessly piles on and crushes hope.

I understood that I was not a visitor from another planet, perhaps the deepest race memory of all if you believe we are stardust, but I still couldn't remember who I was before I woke up in this room, who Marcy was, other than I had a wife and that was her name. I couldn't remember Marcy's face, her voice. All, save the sense memory of her, was gone. Loneliness and a sense of worthlessness weighed on me as memories of Marcy trickled back, and I cried more with each treasured and poisoned gift.

The hospital chaplain was my first visitor. He tried to comfort, to help me to find faith in a divine will. It seemed he had little to say, more likely saw that I was inconsolable. Faith seemed irrelevant when a man killed my wife, and slipped away as I lay dying. I was present at a calamity I couldn't stop and couldn't remember, the chaplain's words forlorn and hopeless. Maybe the existentialists' view of our world would have made more sense right then. Unlike the hospital chaplain's optimistic assurances that God had a plan for me, I might have seen their point.

Existentialists see us confronted by the ever-present necessity to make choices to create our futures. They also point to our tendency to judge and label one another. Their perspective would have helped me face practical truths about my condition, because the harsh limitations imposed on us by those labels can lead to such despair that in his play *No Exit*, Jean-Paul Sartre's character says, "Hell is other people." You can let the judgment of others become your Hell.

Were I capable of forming the thought with my cognitive and memory skills scarcely out of coma, the label others might attach to me was that of a victim imprisoned in his body, one more dead than alive, and—the harshest judgment of all—perhaps better off dead. My body had switched from normal metabolism to catabolism, a destructive process in which the body plunders its stores to release energy. My weight had dropped by perhaps thirty pounds, but there was no way to know what I weighed inside my body cast.

My mother appeared at my bedside. She took my hand and stroked it.

"Simon, in a few days Tamara and the others won't be here at night to help you," she said, her despair so clear to me in the end of day quiet of a hospital, when all the healthy people, who can, have left.

"I'm so sorry. They won't let us keep the private duty nurses."

As I still tried to absorb discovery of Marcy's existence and death, my cocoon of protectors were to be stripped away. In confusion and panic, I pushed my control pad and its precious call button off the edge of my bed. It was the only thing of value I possessed, to push it away my only way to communicate I wanted nothing more to do with this world.

I wanted to roll over and hide from it, hide my tears of despair from my mother. But it took three people to roll me on my side. I could only lie there, the pad dangling by its wire. Three days later, Tamara, Roy, and his entourage were gone, and I faced my first night on my own, with the call button as my only fragile link, confronting a harsh new reality.

Nurse Tamara,
April 6, 1994

Simon Lewis is unable to safely be alone. Memory is affected and unable to use call light for nurses. The patient has also regressed to a childlike stage. This is a high-acute patient.

CHAPTER SEVEN

A HIGH-ACUTE PATIENT

Nights in white satin
Never reaching the end
Letters I've written
Never meaning to send
Beauty I'd always missed
With these eyes before
Just what the truth is
I can't say anymore
                    —Moody Blues,
              "Nights in White Satin"

My first night alone, Marka and Melissa were especially kind, showed me how the call pad was wrapped around the high frame that makes sure hospital patients can't fall out of bed, then disappeared for the night as I watched *Beauty and the Beast* and tried not to panic.

Hell, it turned out, could indeed be other people

when there's no exit. It started with a voice, middle-aged, and a slight European accent: educated and calm.

"Gertrude?" he called, perfectly genial and normal, except it was in the hours between midnight and dawn.

I suddenly wasn't sure if a voice spoke or not. Nobody else on the hospital floor heard or reacted, the ward completely silent. Afraid I'd lost my hold on reality, I listened to the silence.

"Gertrude."

I heard it again, still polite, more insistent, expecting a reply. A longer silence.

Panic welled inside me.

"Gertrooder . . . *telephone!*" the man called. But there was no sound of a phone ringing, and it was long after visiting hours.

With no private duty nurse to help, I needed my call button; anything to stop the voice, now calling every few seconds. It took painful minutes to turn my head until I could see it, and start to creep my fingers across the bed toward that pad and its precious buttons, a distance of perhaps ten inches.

But I couldn't lift my arm when it got there. A child would have known what would happen, but I didn't. When my fingers reached the pad, the rest of my arm pushed it off the edge of my universe, far out of reach.

"Gertroooooooder!!"

The singsong of complete insanity filled my room.

The voice never learned Gertrude wasn't there. It never tired, never grew frustrated or disappointed. I listened to it through the night. When dawn broke, and Karin arrived to start her rounds, I learned my neighbor was once an eminent neurologist, admitted to the rehab floor for one night as a courtesy. He must have loved his wife very much, and carried this memory of her into his afterlife.

By day, Marka and Melissa took care of me. With

the acceptance of a child who never knew a different way, they showed me my special feeding technique. Unable to open my mouth, all food had to be sucked through a big straw. When my mother brought in her home-cooked lasagna, liquefied, I recognized the flavor and became aware of the delicate beauty of taste and smell, and memories of them from my past. Our sense of smell lives in the oldest part of our brain. It's our only sense that physically touches it.

When we visit a place after an absence of many years, it can be its smell that takes us back, through which our minds physically experience the past in a way no photograph can match. That direct contact, the reunion within, is recognized, and our brain responds, "Yes, we were here before."

And that was how good it felt to experience familiar food.

I began to learn from my surroundings, a first, low level of brain function, when a new neighbor entered my consciousness. She was, I learned from her insistent voice, a U.S. mail carrier, whose stroke one day on her mail route changed her life forever. We're accustomed to control of our lives, expect to be asked for our opinion, and play a role in important decisions that affect us and shape our destinies.

Such notions disappear in the whisper of a moment with stroke and brain injury. Through my neighbor, I formed my first conclusion about the unseen world beyond my room, because her reaction to her loss of control was fear that surfaced as anger. I heard it in the way she spoke to the nurses as if they were servants, never asked for something, but ordered it, and never stopped complaining. Her combined fear, frustration, and resentment didn't seem to make any difference to the level of care she received from the nurses, but the easier I made their life, I thought, perhaps the easier they'd make mine. Not very profound, but it was my first conclusion. With the over-compensation that's often a hallmark of brain injury, I became absurdly polite.

Marka and Melissa rounded up a third nurse, often the tireless Karin, to turn me on my side every fifteen minutes to combat bedsores until the arrival of a special inflatable bed. Now they only needed to turn me every twenty minutes, as my new bed huffed and puffed gently to create continual movement under my body. For the first time in my new life, as I listened to my bed through the night, I noticed how there was sound, then the absence of it at the end of each inflation cycle; became aware for the first time of silence. And then I noticed the silence that was inside my head. There was still an absence of inner thought, here at the very bottom of the slope of consciousness, not even the high-pitched, ringing sound called tinnitus, typical of head injury, that would soon become my constant companion.

For now there was the silence of nothingness, an inner emptiness in which there lived no sense of myself, nothing beyond random memories during the day. When night fell, there were no dreams whenever I briefly found sleep; my nights regularly disrupted by nurses as they checked vital signs. Then, one night as I slept, something changed. I still had no sense of my own body, was a mind with no legs and no arms. But I felt a presence nearby, and a fragment memory of a childhood song, in harmony with the presence. The fragment went, "I'm gonna lay down my sword and shield, down by the riverside."

As an image coalesced, I was in a peaceful meadow by a stream, where there sat a knight, arms and head rested on the hilt of his sword, vanquished in battle, silent at my side.

As my brain tried to link pieces of my body, I felt a transition. In my dream, I understood the knight in the meadow was more than my companion. At the moment of transference, I understood that I was the knight, and I felt unutterably cold inside my armor. I couldn't move, not even lift my arm, because it was rusted over, sticky with blood.

> *Down by the riverside*
> *I'm gonna lay my burden down*
> *I ain't gonna trouble the Lord no more*

When I woke from that first dream, my brain wondered about my body, was capable of self-evaluation, and noticed I was unaware of my injuries. My brain had identified something it wanted to understand.

I tried to look at myself, which I never thought of doing before, but could see only my right hand. Bandaged and plastered, cut to the bone by shards of glass, it was drenched with the yellow of iodine. I decided to count my limbs, which also never occurred to me before. It took hours. My hand, I knew, was at the end of one limb, but from my vantage point, that was all of myself I could see. My brain remembered it used to have two arms and two legs.

How many do you have now? it asked.

I didn't know.

How can you tell? it pressed.

I looked at my bandaged right hand, moved its yellowed fingers, and understood. After I counted my fingers several times, it seemed to me that if I started out with four limbs and now could move one, I should figure out the difference. I came to the answer three, and kept repeating it until I understood: three was most of four. For the first time, I understood that almost all of me was hurt.

I cried myself to sleep that night. Trapped in my body, unable to move three of four limbs, with my jaw wired so I could barely eat or speak. I didn't see how things could get any worse.

As the hospital stirred the next day, Melissa came in.

"Good morning, Simon!" she sang brightly, like usual, with her beautiful sunny accent, but there was no response. She looked at me, with open concern, as I looked back, silent.

That night I'd thought about my injuries for the first time, and felt sorry for myself. When I woke, I was sick with a bug, and completely lost my voice. It taught me two lessons. First, that things can always, always, get worse. I vowed at that moment never to feel sorry for myself again, no matter what.

And second, when I woke and realized my predicament, my mind could see the black humor in the loss of my voice, my least damaged link to the world. I grew up with Monty Python on TV, and John Cleese as the Black Knight, who gets each of his limbs chopped off as he insists he'll fight on, until he's only a torso on the ground, still cheerfully undaunted.

"Come back," he challenges, "I'll bite your legs off!"

It's not that I remembered Monty Python or their sketch, but the subconscious connection survived. Whatever parts of me might be dead, the part that made me feel like me, that defined who I was, was still present. It marked another step in the return of my humanity. There was still far to go. Only when doctors removed the cast from my left arm, all of its bone fractures set, did I realize my arm was there. I had only dim awareness of my body, even as nurses removed my catheter. And then there was the bedpan: two nurses to lift me on, two to lift me off. Except one day nobody came back. I pressed the button again, and lay in agony, unable to shout for help. *I have no mouth and I want to scream.*

There was nothing I could do. There are so few

choices when you're a high-acute patient. So I started to count, without purpose, to one hundred. I did that a few times, then fought back panic with a last idea. I began to count backwards from a hundred, as slowly as I could. I didn't know what I'd do when I got to zero this time; the pain was terrible.

I looked up to see David at my door, my savior. Something else struck my brother, as he stood in the door and saw me count backwards. I hadn't reacted; was lost in my own space until he spoke.

"Laddie?" he asked after the nurses cleaned me up. "Look straight ahead, and tell me when you see me."

Easy enough, except I couldn't, not until he stood directly in front of me. My massive right brain injury had completely stripped the left side of my field of vision, another example of the importance of vigilance as the key to recovery: no one diagnosed this problem.

Cedars is a teaching hospital, and high-acute patients make interesting cases for residents, so I was on the guided tour—grand rounds—when the team and its doctors-in-training came by. I didn't know their names, or understand what they said about me, as they stood around my bed and talked.

All the doctors had an opinion. They'd toss ideas back and forth, led by their chief, about what to do with my case, how best to treat me. There was no one else in the room apart from the medical team and me, but I didn't take it personally as doctors ignored me, talked about me in the third person right in front of me as if I wasn't there, because I didn't feel as if I was in the room either.

I didn't understand my existence, let alone my role as patient, but I did focus on every word of one physician, Doctor Blue Eyes. It wasn't anything he said; it never occurred to me to listen to that, but because his eyes were so blue. They fascinated me, but it was another doctor one week, who stayed as the rest walked on.

"Good morning, Mr. Lewis . . . ," he started slow-ly, the first doctor to speak to me in my new life.

I heard this man I didn't know say my name, and felt surprised and confused.

"My name is Dr. John Croft . . . ," he prompted, and then waited for his patient to respond.

Except I didn't understand that I was supposed to answer. A doctor with compassion, he wasn't discour-aged by my blank silence and guessed what he must do to connect with me, to enter my world.

He gently took my right hand, the first person other than my parents to make physical contact in so long. I responded to the warmth, felt it enter my inner world, and looked up to his eyes.

"Courage," he said simply, and planted that sin-gle word there.

He patted the back of my hand three times; each stirred echoes in my mind. I was so grateful for the hu-man contact.

"*Courage*," he said softly one last time, and left to rejoin his group. And I understood that doctors who talked about me could also talk *to* me.

I thought about his one word for days. I knew that I was hurt, but not really why I needed courage, and wondered if the doctor knew I wasn't a brave person.

Slowly, it occurred to me that if he'd spoken to me, I could ask him. He only came once a week, and I was ready for his next visit with the only question I could think of, the one answer I needed most.

"You said, 'Have courage,'" I whispered through wired teeth, grateful when he took my hand again.

"I don't know if I have any, or where to find it."

Dr. Croft smiled.

"For some people, Simon, the decision to open their eyes in the morning . . . is an act of courage."

CHAPTER EIGHT

MEANING

"Beauty is truth, truth beauty—that is all
You know on earth, and all you need to know."
—John Keats,
"Ode on a Grecian Urn"

I'm not a brave man, and my path to full recovery didn't begin with a bold, courageous choice. At least, it didn't seem that way when doctors confirmed my sutures—the scarlet patchwork quilt of incisions on my head, hand, abdomen, hip and pelvis—were clean and secure, and a physical therapist, whose name was Luke, came to move me through a simplified range of motion every four hours. Because my pelvis was still unable to support me upright, I had to be kept horizontal at all times. I learned this one day when Melissa, Marka, Karin, and Luke all gathered in my room at the same time.

"Magic carpet!" Marka called out of my room. More helpers soon gathered in response around my bed, and each grabbed hold of my home—the sheet I lay on. I could feel them tug on my limbs as they took up the slack. I couldn't remember when I was this closely sur-rounded by so many nurses and therapists, so many hands laid on me at the same time.

"Relax, hon," Marka reassured.

My body went rigid with fear.

"One . . . two . . . three!"

On "three," my broken body felt the sheet pull hard against it and, for the briefest moment, overcome gravity as they heaved it into the air. A second later, my carcass landed like a sack of potatoes on the ready gur-ney, and Marka sped me on my first ceiling-tile tour of the hospital (for that's all I could see of it) into my first MRI, as doctors evaluated me head to foot.

In time, I'd call the gap between what doctors' evaluations could tell me and I needed to know "the Mantra." It goes along the lines of, "We don't know whether you'll improve, and if you do, there's no way to know how much." The Brain Injury Association of America's website warns every visitor who needs defi-nite answers that, "prevention is the only known cure for brain injury."

With the limitations of my treatment and likely recovery officially recognized, it fell to Dr. Coulton, a young ginger-haired doctor-in-training, to conduct my psychological evaluation.

"Good morning, Mr. Lewis," he introduced him-self, courteous and a little formal in his white coat. He confirmed I knew who and where I was, and ran tests until I was too tired to continue. Then, perhaps as in-structed by his medical school professors, to encourage the patient and establish a relationship of trust, he leaned in close as our first session ended.

"It's difficult for you to come to terms with this now . . . ," he began seriously, and then brightened. "But you'll look back one day, and see how this experience made you a better, stronger person!"

I wasn't capable of anger yet, only of utter, bewildered shock. He just told me my wife's senseless murder made me a better person; the New Age folklore that somehow everything happens for the best, when it doesn't. That's why it's a tragedy.

My parents confronted Coulton later and gave it to him straight.

"We hope one day *your* wife dies this way and someone tells *you* it's for the best."

He apologized profusely, and it was a while before I saw him again. Instead, a speech and language pathologist began to test my ability to express and receive words, a kindly older woman I met again years later and learned was Ellen DeGeneres's mother. She was quiet, gentle, and understanding, as she asked me to pick the odd one out from a list. Was it cloud, rain, snow, fog, or car?

I struggled to remember what they were as she tested whether my ability to reason logically was compromised. From my simple perspective, the effort to remember these objects, and her other tests that referenced the outside world I'd lost, led me to another question.

John Croft was back in my room on his weekly grand rounds. Only one question mattered, and it had never occurred to me before.

"Doctor, how long do I have to live?"

I was curious, but not worried about John's answer. I didn't feel present or alive, so would accept it calmly if he told me only a few days remained.

"Hard to say," he replied, "your internal systems are healing, so you may have years ahead of you."

I couldn't remember having lived a whole year, but knew it was a long time. And as if to confirm Croft's opinion, at the end of April, another flying carpet ride took me to get images of my jaw fractures, which showed they had fused. A few days later, Dr. Anderson appeared in my room.

"Time to unwire your jaw," he murmured, X-rays held to the light.

As I thought how nice it might be to eat some way other than liquid sucked through a straw, Anderson wrapped one hand around my head in a wrestler's lock, a pair of pliers appeared in his other from a pocket, and he yanked hard on my jaw, until blood spurted in my mouth and I went into shock at this dentistry from the Middle Ages. He stuck one of my fingers between my teeth when he was done, to show how my jaw could open.

"Increase to three fingers over the next few days," he prescribed, and was gone.

I lay there, too weak to call a nurse to change my bloodstained sheets, until Marka spotted me.

"What happened to *you* honey?" There was no answer.

"Doctor was here?"

A weak nod.

"Didn't he medicate you?"

I managed a weak shake.

"Those wires went through your bone," her voice rose in anger. "If I'd *known* he was comin' today I woulda premedicated you. Why didn't he *tell* me?"

I heard her indignation, but no longer cared about the hospital's lack of communication: I could put my forefinger between my teeth. I could open my mouth.

A little later, Melissa stopped in to cheer me up. One effect of being bedridden for weeks on end is you become part of the life of the hospital, and Melissa had confided she'd started to date a doctor. On her way to the door she paused, then turned.

"Do *you* think I look like a cock-a-roach?" she asked.

It was the first time in my new life that someone asked for my opinion, and it felt very nice. I looked at her cute, petite body and inquiring smile, and considered carefully whether she looked like a roach.

"Um, I don't think so," I said.

And for the first time since the crash, I could open my mouth to speak, and to smile. It felt so nice that another instinctive question rose to my lips.

"Why do you ask?"

"Because my boyfriend says I do with my hair this way."

Then she bobbed her head to one side, and I got it. She'd colored her hair chocolate brown with a home kit, and her front fringe was spiked up with mousse into little pointies. When she bobbed her head like that, they sort of quivered like little brown antenna.

"I'm not sure what he means, but maybe you should make him happy and try a different style?"

As always, Melissa's beauty and smile cheered me. Luke began to advance my basic physical therapy to cope with the essential activities of daily living, or ADLs. It took time to advance from how to roll me over onto one side and back with carefully timed assistance from Luke and two nurses, to the point they could lift my body up to a sitting position on the edge of my bed. I was still unable to stand, but it felt special to sit upright, if only for a few seconds, before nurses laid me back down.

Dr. Coulton appeared again at my bedside and moved me on to more tests. Shapes to study, then try to draw from memory, blocks to move around a board in the right sequence. He seemed more interested in me, though it never occurred to me to ask him why. Perhaps he despaired whether I would ever ask him anything.

"Simon," he said one day, after I struggled through his session, "you know when a football player gets knocked unconscious, and the coaches run up? They always ask three questions as soon as he opens his eyes: 'What's your name?' 'Where are you?' and 'What year is this?'"

I gazed at him attentively, a bit confused. "Huh, interesting," I managed, and then fell silent after my noncommittal comment.

"So much brain damage can occur after he's out cold on the field for those few seconds—what we call a *mild* injury to it—they have to check," Dr. Coulton pressed ahead. "Now, *moderate* injury is the damage the brain suffers when someone is unconscious *for more than twenty minutes. . . .*"

Maybe he hoped I'd offer another comment, but nothing crossed my mind. He had no choice but to go on.

"*Severe* brain injury, Simon, is what happens to it after six hours of coma. . . ."

There was still no reaction.

"*Massive* brain injury," he continued, his voice tinged with sad resignation, "is thought to occur after loss of consciousness *for one week.*"

As if to prove his worst fears, my face showed no sign I'd any idea where this might lead. I didn't. It simply sounded interesting, in a distant way.

"Simon," he finished, "you were in coma *for a month.*"

Nothing prepared me for the implications of Coulton's final words, that my mind was too damaged to recover, my detachment from the normal world would not end. I'd yet to come to terms with Marcy's death, and now learned I might also never be reunited with the person I once was. Marcy, and the man beside her, were both gone.

Dr. Coulton watched my reaction closely and urgently reported it to my parents, with whom he'd now built a good relationship.

"I need you to authorize visitors immediately," he advised, "or we'll lose him."

The first to appear in my room the next morning were my brother David and his wife Lilly with their six-year-old twins Nikki and Jason, led by their eight-year-old sister Stephanie in full Native American costume and makeup. All three of their kids jumped at the chance to visit because, if Uncle Simon couldn't come to their school musical, *Pippin*, they could bring the show to me.

Nikki loved to sing and dance. Costumed and face-painted as a cat, with the voice of a little angel, she led her twin brother Jason, who was costumed as the little boy from the show and still clutching his character's stuffed pet duck, Otto, the two clearly inseparable.

With Stephanie, they jumped and careened through my tiny room, impervious to all except the sunshine of youth and life. They made gleeful little bows for a perfect finale. With my spirits lifted, other hints of the outside world now gradually came through the door. One of the hardships of head injury is that in a thirty-minute visit friends don't realize how the victim's life has changed. Mine saw my bare scalp—its long horseshoe scar line visible on my shaved head, the bandages and bruises—but also saw who they believed was their "same old Simon."

It creates its own set of problems for stroke and head-trauma victims, who often suffer repeat head injuries, as friends, family, insurance companies and victims alike embrace a mistaken notion that they are ready to resume normal activities. My parents wisely started with friends who'd reinforce my fractured identity.

Howie Mandel visited Cedars the day after the media identified me. Visitors aren't allowed into the ICU—access is strictly limited—but Cedars always made stars welcome. In the midst of tragedy, my parents looked up one night to see Howie standing there. He saw the evening news, came straight in to help and now, two months later, we talked about past and future, how show business is like a traveling band of players who come together, whether to produce another show or in time of crisis. Howie wanted me to know that he was there for me, whenever I was ready.

There was Ronnie Rubin, who ran the Department of the Arts at UCLA Extension, where I taught before I was an adjunct professor at USC. A great friend through the years, she brought me a book of Van Gogh pictures. I couldn't hold the book when Ronnie showed it to me, let alone read it, but there were to be times when in the dead hours between midnight and dawn I'd find comfort in Van Gogh's swirling clouds of dazzling, thick-layered colors, of beauty in agony.

Joy and Harvey were eager to see me again after the terrible crash they witnessed, and Tova, who flew from Italy for our wedding and returned for Marcy's funeral, came down from her San Francisco home, but saw I was not ready to talk about her final service for her best friend.

Keith Gordon, the director, and Bob Weide, the writer-producer of *Mother Night*, came together and said Nick Nolte loved our screenplay and had agreed to star. The movie would go into production as soon as they finished the rest of casting. I congratulated them with all my heart, but it was hard to feel another piece of my life slip away, for no one knew if I would ever again be on the set of a movie I brought to life.

Finally Marcy's parents flew in, and we wept for their only child who was gone. I asked her father if the crash was my fault, as none of my visitors told me what happened. No, he said, there was no way anyone could have seen the truck coming, and no one stopped the driver as he ran away. There's no closure in real life.

At the end of each visit, my kind visitors walked out into a world of activity I could no longer remember or imagine and I remained bedridden, exhausted by the effort of conversation and communication, in my world of doctors' evaluations. The medical chart that hung from the foot of my bed fairly burst with all manner of information, but the real, and much deeper meaning I sought, the central ambiguity of my new life that remained unanswered by my doctors, was whether or how I'd ever again interact with that world outside my door.

My personal and professional friends confronted me with unanswerable questions. I'd defined myself all my working life by what I accomplished alongside them. Now I was forced to ask myself who I was *without* any of those projects and pastimes; and to question my role and my meaning in the world if I had no goals. The most obvious and immediate one—to prepare for the day I could leave Cedars—never occurred to me. Before my visitors, the foreign universe outside my room was beyond my imagination and it still never crossed my mind that I might one day leave either the room in which I lay, or the hospital. The more I tried to think of one, the more I came back to only one task, one goal that I might accomplish. It was to never let my family see me despair.

This would, I knew, be a comfort to them and my only way to give thanks for all their love and support. But if I accepted a future with no goals beside inner acceptance of my condition and outward optimism, I couldn't see the meaning to my life. A lovely physical therapist would help me find it, the entrance to the hidden path, as I approached a critical threshold. Another grand rounds conference was held around my bed, half a dozen doctors, plus nurses and therapists, with a brief summary in my chart: "Doing well. Stein to do EMG nerve conduction study. . . . Jaw position good. . . . Electric stim. to left arm."

The key test was Dr. Norman Stein's EMG, to insert needles and watch my nerves react. After the precisely induced and measured pain, his report was filled with his tentative findings, language that relied on phrases like *"tend to favor"* and *"suggesting* intact nerve function." It was an early sign of how little doctors could tell me about my peripheral nerves and my brain or, for that matter, what the future held for either.

That week, the team wheeled my gurney to a Memorial Day party at Cedars, two years since the holiday weekend in Lake Tahoe when I first met Marcy and found the most complete happiness of my life.

Memorial Day held special memories that I could never again share with my wife, and that made me feel very lonely as I participated in the celebration with my family, caregivers, and fellow-patients. But Dr. Stein's tentatively positive findings marked my passage across the threshold to full inpatient therapy on a daily basis.

Tina, a young and beautiful dark-haired woman with skill and kindness in equal measure, began intensive sessions to mobilize my arms, head, and neck to the point that I could, with the use of one arm, roll myself onto my side and back. In her transfer program, she explained how with practice I might move my body from bed to chair, and I could scarcely believe it when the day came and, my right arm clasped around Tina for support, I transferred myself off my bed.

No medical report could describe what it felt like to sit on a chair for the first time in three months, see my room from a different perspective than horizontal, my head held high. From my new vantage point, I looked up at Tina gratefully, then stared down at my left leg, a confused animal that knew the leg once belonged to me, but with no sense it was lost, because paralysis means you can't feel it's not there—you don't even feel its absence. While I sat, therapists attached the electrodes that Stein prescribed to my left arm.

It was my first introduction to electrical stimulation and I looked in wonder when I saw my left arm move, but felt nothing as it stirred for the first time.

"Reach out," Tina prompted, and I watched my arm reach. I didn't know whether it was the electricity or me that made it happen, why an arm that hung limply from my left shoulder moved at her command.

Because Tina could safely get me into a chair she could also take me to the next transfer level: to a wheelchair. Out through my door she wheeled me, further beyond it than I could see from my bed, into what looked like another dimension.

Unlike the ceiling-tile tours on my gurney rides, I could turn my head as Tina pushed me in the wheelchair, and look at the world right side up. I was surprised to see Marka at a nurse's station smile and wave, to see she existed outside my room. With no understanding of what lay beyond the strip of carpet at my visual borderline, everything here was unexpected, most of all our destination—the hospital gym, a room filled with equipment and floor-to-ceiling windows, with a view of the Los Angeles hills.

"Simon, say hi to Bert!" Tina introduced me.

She'd wheeled me up to the hospital skeleton—Bert—for a guided tour of my injuries. There are two hundred and six bones in your body, and it looked like I'd broken most of the big ones, but not my back.

"Even your fractures have fractures," Tina explained sorrowfully, as one by one she pointed out broken ribs and other bones. She transferred me from the wheelchair onto a pallet, very carefully so that no weight was put on my legs, and began.

Every culture gives pain a different meaning and

place, an expectation of how that society expects its members to cope with it. I'd grown up with the British stiff upper lip approach, which is to greet pain with humor. "Does it hurt, Sergeant?" the officer asks the mortally wounded soldier.

"Only when I laugh, sir," the dying man replies.

That sort of stuff.

I lay there, fascinated by the sunlight streaming through the windows and the dappled beauty of the Los Angeles hills I could see through them, surrounded by delightful, caring therapists, many of them fit and very attractive young women like Tina. They and their beauty disappeared, along with all reserve and stiff upper lip learned since childhood, as my back arched, my head threw back, and I bellowed in animalistic agony.

Without warning, Tina had slowly, mind-bendingly crossed my legs, mobilizing my pelvis after months, which tore into groin and bowels. Then she uncrossed them, which didn't hurt so much, because I fainted. My pelvis had set, another milestone.

It's an intimate relationship between physical therapist and patient, and Tina could sense from my lack of response during her session that I hadn't connected Bert or the gym with my body. More and more, I was preoccupied with the questions my visitors provoked, about where, ultimately, my recovery was headed. Of what I was now and what would become of me, of what meaning my life had at this point, if everything that gave meaning to it was gone.

Soon after, Dr. Almendros introduced himself in my room. From my limited view of the world, this amiable doctor in his white coat seemed to spring from nowhere. He asked me about myself.

"I don't know who I am," I told him truthfully, "or where I'm going."

He diagnosed that I suffered from anxiety.

"Would you like me to put you on Buspar for that?" he asked.

I was never one to take pills unless absolutely necessary.

"Are there side effects, Doctor?"

"Nothing much." Almendros hesitated. "You may feel somnolent—sleepy—but that's about it. Here. . . ." He scribbled on a pad his prescription to take away anxiety.

The Buspar pills did relax me as I took them that day. I felt no anxiety at all by next morning as I looked out my window, entranced as always by the light. Somehow, everything seemed especially peaceful. Then I felt my mind and body lift gently, up and up, and hover over the bed.

It was beautiful to be free; I looked down on myself, at my broken bedridden body where it lay, considered myself and what I had become, and slowly, in tranquility, passed through, beyond my window, into the light. Then softly, with acceptance and understanding, made a gentle decision to return and reclaim my body. Borne by a sunbeam on glittering motes of dust.

When she visited, my mother thought she detected a change. It was difficult to tell for sure because I remained so distant, so withdrawn from my visitors. But now, when she looked in my eyes, she thought I was absent, that Elvis had left the building. Dr. Almendros assessed me, prescribed Buspar and moved on, but the drug's side effects were not limited to somnolence as he claimed. I was stoned out of my damaged mind, and there was a risk of seizures if I stopped my fix. Saved once again by their vigilance, my family overcame resistance from the medical team, who gradually weaned me off. Mercifully, I never suffered seizures when they did.

Perhaps tripping out did help me find meaning in life, because it was while on Buspar that Tina wheeled me into the hospital lobby to a little birdcage set into the wall, which was atwitter with tiny, brightly colored birds. It was the poet William Blake who asked, "How can the bird that is born for joy sit in a cage and sing?"

Well, these miniature birds in their habitat set into a wall at Cedars-Sinai, deprived of flight, and almost everything else a bird might normally expect from life, chirped away as happy as can be. As I looked, I felt I understood why the caged bird sings.

I looked, and thought I heard them sing to me, "Simon, I know I can't fly, but isn't it so great to be here!"

It was. I realized my ability to perceive these birds and them to see me, was one of the most beautiful facts of life. I began to appreciate my own existence, and when I got back to my room I lay there, awed by the uniqueness of perception and awareness—the ability to see and hear the little songbirds, appreciate flavors and smells, and experience beauty in all its forms.

Gradually, with electrical stimulation, more strength flowed into my left arm. As sensation and control returned, Tina showed me how I could push my wheelchair myself. The day arrived that a fresh set of X-rays confirmed my pelvis was set long enough to attempt for it to bear my weight. Tina wheeled me to a different gym, one with low parallel bars.

"Nose over your toes, and stand," she instructed, as she guided my two hands onto the support rails.

I tried, uncertainly, to tighten my leg muscles, and nothing happened. When a peripheral nerve to a muscle is severed, the muscle becomes limp. When nerve fibers in the brain or spinal cord are damaged, the tone of some muscles may become increased, and they resist being stretched—a condition called spasticity. With both peripheral and central nerve injuries, and after all the trauma and months of inactivity, my muscles could do nothing. Then gradually, haltingly, they responded to different degrees. And as I painfully stood for the first time, naked in my hospital gown, I started to weep, not for joy, nor out of grief. I wept because I was unable to cope with the feelings and memories that flooded me.

"Take a step," Tina murmured. And my limp left leg dragged forward, hands grasped on the bars, as tears streamed. Behind me, another therapist calmly called "Code Blue," for her patient a few feet away, a death alert that required immediate help from every nurse in the unit. A vacuum formed around me, as I clung to my parallel bars. While I struggled to stay upright, there were unmistakable sounds of a defibrillator, a quiet hiss as the Code Blue team started oxygen and established IV access. I felt stranded, washed up on the uncertain borderline between a life and a death; between an alert, oriented patient and one without pulse or respiration. I'd never know the outcome as the team wheeled Code Blue away, whether his path that morning led back to life, a physician, and a family, or to a coroner with a death certificate. And I felt ashamed to weep, merely because I stood up. I was back in my wheelchair, desperate to retreat to my room, but Tina wanted to calm me.

"I expected you to cry, Simon," she said. "Many patients do when they take their first step. Let's go outside."

Before I could panic, Tina wheeled me past a decorative waterfall into the hospital courtyard. I'd forgotten what it felt like to physically move through a wide, open, space, an experience beyond imagination in my bed. I felt the sun on my face, felt wind stir my hair. There's no wind indoors. I'd forgotten about that, too.

Perhaps it was tripping out on Buspar that first pointed me toward the way back, that started me on the path to find meaning in the world I drifted out to join through the window during my out-of-body experience.

A Code Blue patient at the edge of life, birds sing-
ing in a cage, and my first taste of a world glimpsed
through gym windows. They were fleeting moments of
pain and healing, of death and beauty: the agony and
ecstasy of life. Perhaps these experiences gave me the
courage Dr. Croft said I needed to find the hidden path.
To believe there could be a pattern and meaning in my
life even now.

And above all else, I began to absorb that there
was a world, *outside.*

CHAPTER NINE

FEAR, AND HOPE

Mine is the last voice that you will ever hear . . .
Don't be alarmed. . . .
—Frankie Goes to Hollywood,
"Two Tribes"

I saw it when Tina wheeled me back, and helped transfer me onto my bed. A calendar was neatly hung on the wall below the clock. It was June 7 and, Karin told me, my discharge was set for the fourteenth.

When doctors use the word "crisis," they mean the time when their patient either dies, or starts to recover. If the calendar marked the end of my medical crisis as far as they were concerned, it was the start of a personal one for me. For it slowly sank in that discharge meant I would go home; and I still couldn't recall anything about it. I tried to remember, and slowly recalled flagstones on a garden path that led to a front door with shiny black studs and lay in my bed, satis-

fied. As I stared at my discharge date, I began to grasp
that however weak, vulnerable, and unprepared I was,
what I faced was not a crisis, which is in every sense
negative, but my future—the life that remained to me
in the blank pages of that calendar, which was positive,
if unknown.

There's a Chinese pictograph that can either
mean crisis or opportunity, the Zen symbol for life's
paradox. Now was my moment to choose for those un-
written months ahead, between fear and hope; to be a
victim, or a survivor. I didn't understand why Cedars
set a date with recovery barely begun but I tried, like
the producer I once was, to prepare myself for an outside world I saw in the courtyard one time. Except I'd
no idea how to overcome my fears in the days that remained, or where on earth to find the courage to go on,
like Dr. Croft urged. I asked myself hard questions;
whether I wanted in my heart to recover, when all I
held most precious was lost. I wasn't sure, and began
to cry again. More questions followed: if I didn't want
to recover, whether I wanted instead to close my eyes
and give up. That seemed the only choice I had. Go on,
or give up. If I gave up, I couldn't imagine what would
happen next, nor, if I decided to go on, any sense of what
recovery could accomplish.

I'd no idea how to answer that question. My brain
wasn't yet capable to make a decision, even of whether
I wanted to recover, and I had one week left before discharge.

I knew for sure it was my decision alone, my responsibility to achieve recovery, only because I over-
heard a doctor in the next room joke to a colleague about
his patient.

"He said to me, 'Doctor, it's *your job* to *make* me
better!' Can you believe that?!"

The two of them had a good laugh about how ridiculous this patient's notion was.

So that question at least was answered. Only I could choose. I struggled with my fear for hours, as I stared at my blank white hospital door, and all the unseen uncertainty that lay beyond it. Gradually I saw that my life, my future, and my recovery, were a hallway, like the one I occasionally glimpsed over the shoulders of my visitors when they came in through that door.

We all enter the world through a door at one end, and as we walk down the long hallway of our life, we see an infinite number of doors off it that we can go through. Each door leads to rooms and more doors inside, but always we will return to the hallway, as the years advance, and we change with them. Some doors lead to rooms that are empty, some filled with grief, still others with profound happiness, the greatest treasure hunt on earth. At the end is the final door, through which we must all pass, and we want to find and enjoy as many of the treasures of life as we can before we reach it. The hallway was still there for me, as solid as that first white door before my eyes. There was still, I realized, a path of recovery to explore, the path every victim must find, and discharge meant the time approached when I must find mine.

At first I felt terribly alone. I knew in one sense our journey through life is solitary, for we are born alone and we die alone, leave the earth as simply as we arrive, when our path takes us to that final door. And then I realized that, in some of the most important senses of all, I wasn't alone.

There was my loving family, who sustained and supported me every day both in my first life and my new one, and a dawning realization that we stand on the shoulders of those who came before. On my side biologically were thousands of generations who, for me to have survived, all maximized their healing, and their lives;

nurtured my capacity to recover. Their timeless contribution was their gift to me, not only for physical healing, but emotionally, in the circuits and systems that shaped my consciousness and guided my decisions. But the question remained of whether, at the age of thirty-six, it was too late to start over, of what kind of performance, what level of recovery, my brain was still capable.

With so much uncertainty about my future, I made a choice that gave me hope. I'd believe there was a path to full recovery. I didn't know, any more than my doctors, who couldn't say if such a path existed. And if it did, it was totally hidden from sight. But I felt that not to seek it with all the strength I could muster made failure certain; that to succeed I must commit myself to the search, and make the best decisions I could, one baby choice at a time.

To make the right choices would be hard. My brain couldn't tell me if any plans I made were the right ones, or realistic. Nor for that matter, even if it could gradually heal, could my brain step outside of itself, look back, and assess progress. And if it couldn't, I wondered how I'd know if I improved. A childhood memory surfaced, of a science fiction story I read. There were these scientists at a test center who experimented with time travel. They'd go, then come back and see what was different. But whatever they tried, nothing changed. As far as the scientists could tell, nothing worked.

Except at the beginning, they were in a state of the art laboratory, and by the end of the story they were in an empty cave. In the last chapter, the scientists declared the time-travel experiment a failure. As they dismantled their civilization, they'd changed everything but didn't know, because they'd no way to measure it.

Making the best decisions to recover my brain seemed the same, with no way to measure myself except a badly broken yardstick that could remember no more of my home than the path to its front door. I tried to stay calm as I contemplated my future after discharge, before I remembered where my parents would take me when I left this hospital room, or had answers to most of my questions. As my final days at Cedars closed in, Dr. Croft visited on his rounds, and I told him my fears.

"Healing your brain may take five years, or longer," he explained. "You need to stay close with those who will wait for you, Simon. Otherwise, by the time you're ready to return to life, your friends may have moved on."

After several cancellations, Tina was finally able to book a specially equipped ambulance with an elevator to lift my wheelchair on board, and take me to a nearby pool for what was to be my only visit for water therapy.

As a device that seemed to date from the Civil War shakily lowered me, seated, into the water, and I submerged and felt my limp body float weightless, I still wondered many things. Like Peggy Lee sighs in her song of disillusionment, "Is that all there is . . . Is that all there is?"

I wondered how much further I could recover, with my time at Cedars all but gone.

My family felt the pressure of time in a different way. They witnessed my one trip for water therapy, and what it took to transport me there. They were ready to help in any way possible, but weren't foolhardy. I clearly wasn't in any shape to come home, obvious to all except the insurer. From its point of view, my approved healing times were up, and therefore I was ready. Time pressure grew daily. A folding walker, a frame you move in front while you support yourself with your arms, was approved though I wasn't yet able to use one, as well as a wheelchair, to ready me for discharge. The freight train accelerated, even if it had no driver, and it seemed regardless of the facts of my medical condition. Once again my parents became advocates.

"How will he get in the car to come home?" my father argued strenuously with Pauline Rossi, my Catastrophic Case Manager. If I couldn't make that first transfer, I couldn't continue my recovery as an outpatient. He insisted I not be discharged until I was capable of unassisted transfer into a car, and won me one extra week at Cedars. At $2,000 a day for my room, plus everything I received there, Great-West earned its name again.

The news of a one-week reprieve lifted my spirits. I didn't know schedules could change, that more time could be found for recovery if there was a good reason. And in that grace period, I finally found a reason, and hope, to go on.

I found them in Marcy's memory. Had I died, and Marcy survived, I'd want her to make the most of her future without me. The same immutable truth applied to us both: life must be lived by the living. It was my first decision to embrace my new life, and the plan I made to do that was some day, any day, to walk one hundred yards, unaided by handrails or anything else. On that day, if my left leg collapsed, I promised myself that I'd crawl back, if necessary on my stomach with my right arm, and that would make two hundred.

I knew my plan was incomplete, but it was the only one I could think of. Even as it left all the unanswered questions about how to find a path to recovery to simple hope, all my therapies accelerated and everything about me began to happen too soon.

I knew time would always be a problem. I could see it in the rush of final tests crammed into the end of a three-and-a-half-month hospital stay. I was wheeled down to Dr. Anderson for a comprehensive acoustic test. Amidst all the uncertainty about my future, my hearing was intact. Three tiny eardrum bones—the small-est in the human body, no bigger than a grasshopper's legs—survived the crushing of my skull. It was proof of the miraculous design of our bodies that gives the high-est protection to our most vital organs. My pelvis, ribs, and skull fulfilled their evolutionary mission, as they were pushed to the point of failure, yet preserved my life within.

Dr. Coulton came by for a farewell visit. We'd be-come quite friendly, and he wanted to impress one fact on me.

"Listen very carefully," he said. "In the years ahead, you'll be given a lot of wrong information about your lost vision. Doctors will tell you that it's a *cut*, and there's nothing to be done. But I've done many subtle tests on you, and it's a *neglect*. There's always the pos-sibility it may improve."

He wanted to give me a scientific basis for opti-mism, and though I didn't understand what he said, I understood what he meant: that there was hope for my vision. And when two Intensive Care nurses came by to introduce themselves as sisters, who together nursed me through my coma, they recommended I make an ap-pointment as soon as possible with Dr. Alan Brodney, a leading vision specialist in L.A.

ICU patients can't remember their critical care nurses, which makes these lifesavers the kindest-heart-ed caregivers of all, and it was wonderful to meet and give thanks to two of mine.

Dr. Voight, which I discovered was the name of the doctor who led all the others in those weekly grand rounds, provided the written referral to Dr. Brodney, and described my "amazingly good progress during re-habilitation." My parents innocently mentioned they'd bring champagne on my last day, and he set them straight.

"Simon's brain injury is beyond massive," he explained in our final family conference. "He needs to try and grow new neurons, but alcohol dissolves them. It would be like planting seeds, then pouring gasoline on top to make them grow."

It was a literally sobering thought, and a sign of how little my family was told to expect for my future. The day before discharge, I was taken out for a farewell lunch by Tina, Luke, and Jean, my key therapists, to an Italian restaurant next door to Cedars. It was my first time on a sidewalk, first time in a public restaurant. As a producer, I seemed to live there, in meetings with executives, agents, and talent. Now I was there in a cotton smock with an IV connector still on the back of my hand.

Tina, who brought me through so much with unmatchable kindness, gave me a book she found in a bookstore, and kept for the day I would return to the outside world.

It was called *Simon's Night*—she had bought it for me as soon as she read the cover, which described it as "the highly praised story of one man's determination to get the most out of life."

It felt so strange to be outside in the world with my therapists, before the last night of my long stay at Cedars. But as that final evening drew on, I lay in my hospital bed, read the cover of Tina's gift, and knew that like my namesake character in the book, I too had found the faith, and had a plan, to try and get the most out of life.

It was June 13, 1994, the same night that Nicole Brown Simpson's dog would lead neighbors to the double murder scene of her and Ron Goldman that occurred the previous night, where blood flowed, "like a river."

While so many other tragedies played out, I woke up the next morning to the discharge paperwork. As a head injury patient improves, doctors use a Rancho Los Amigos Scale to track progress. That scale runs from 1 (no response to stimuli) up to 8 (purposeful and oriented, with appropriate recall and behavior).

The "amazingly good progress" Dr. Voight described was that the Cedars team advanced me from level 1 to level 6, which meant that I had a beginning awareness of my own self and others, with multiple physical impairments, but I also understood very little, didn't connect the absence of champagne as a clue to my future, that no one would discuss.

One person who wondered about my future was Dr. Richard Van Allan, the interventional radiologist who came out late that night in March to help save my life. He asked, and was told that "the patient walked out of the hospital." Case closed.

CHAPTER TEN

HOME

*In three words I can sum up everything I've
learned about life: it goes on.*
                                    —Robert Frost

From my parents' perspectives, "walked" was no way
to describe how their son left Cedars. In the real
world, rather than the one in medical records, my
parents stood at the curb of the hospital's drive-through
pickup zone, and discussed how to squeeze my almost
rigid body into their sedan with an overworked intern
who wheeled me there. It was tricky. Whatever they
tried, one or another of my limbs wouldn't fit. The answer they hit on was to slide the front passenger seat
all the way back, and recline it to near horizontal. The
intern lifted me from the curbside wheelchair, and then
lowered me in.

Liberated from my IV and hospital ID bracelet
after so long, I heard the busy morning traffic as our car

pulled away from Cedars, and watched glimpses of palm trees pass in the bright sunshine, until I fell asleep.

When we arrived, there was no flagstone pathway, or studded front door. Only then did I realize that this image was of my childhood home in Wimbledon, England. This home in front of me was my parents' comfortable ranch-style house, on a quiet residential road in the San Fernando Valley.

It was mid-afternoon, and my bedroom was ready. A constant red glow emanated from next to the bed.

"Simon's not used to the dark," Luke warned, and recommended a night lamp so I wouldn't get scared, after months in hospital where it's never dark or quiet.

It felt so nice in the crisp sheets of a regular bed. Welcome memories returned, of when my parents and brothers agreed on this house after we arrived in California, a good location from which to find work in our new city and country. My parents created a warm and loving home here and over the years, my brothers and I bought homes of our own. As shadows lengthened and dusk came on, I listened to my parents' TV in the living room, comforted by what I saw around me in the warm beam of my night light.

Morning brought my first challenge: I couldn't move. A hospital bed has side rails, which I relied on at Cedars to raise myself to a sitting position. I followed the steps Tina taught me: moved fingers first, then wrists, to gradually unlock every one of my internal and external scars frozen solid during the night. In a regular bed with no side rails, it took a full hour just to swing my legs over and sit up. When, finally, I perched on the edge of my bed ready to transfer my weight, I wanted to chirp for joy, just like the birds outside my window. It fell to my mother to help me bathe and dress for my first outpatient care, provided in a building that looked like a converted office block. Dr. Whitney, a pleasant man with a round face who, as head of Cedars outpatient rehab, would supervise my case, met me in his office. He had a model of a head on his desk, and cradled it in delicate hands.

"When there's a blow to the head, we call it a 'coup.'"

He pointed at the skull in a redundant gesture.

"The brain sits in fluid, so the shock travels *through* the brain until it hits the other side of the skull and suffers more damage, which we call the 'contrecoup.'"

So that was it: two insults to the brain from one blow.

"The nerves cross over," Whitney continued, "so we think the right brain damage is why your left body is so weak."

I waited for more, but he was done, apart from perfunctory confirmation of my paperwork. It was therapy time, but far from a brave new world of the intensive and more advanced recovery I hoped for and needed, there was a forty-minute session of brainteasers, a little physical therapy, and I was finished for the day. Twice each week, I showed up at the office building, met a physical therapist in a gym on the ground floor, then rode up in the elevator to the ninth floor, where, because the hospital couldn't schedule consecutive appointments, I slept on a cot until another round of brain teasers. There was plenty of down time to consider his words before my next appointment with Dr. Whitney, because it wasn't until a month later.

"You said the right brain makes my left body work?" I asked him, once again in his office. He nodded politely.

"Does that mean, if I do everything with my left hand, that it will force my right brain to try harder?"

"It might."

"Will it harm me if I try?" I puzzled, unclear of

his advice.

"I don't think so," Whitney reflected.

He didn't intend to be unhelpful, though my questions seemed so obvious and easy that I hesitated to ask them. But as Whitney thought my idea wouldn't harm me, I tried to eat and drink, shave and brush my teeth, with only my left hand.

There were follow-ups with other doctors too, such as my first visit as an outpatient to Dr. Brien, the surgeon who rebuilt my body with titanium hardware in his twelve-hour marathon. He was one of the many doctors who saved my life. But Brien didn't seem that interested to see me again, even though my pelvis was frozen. I could move only inches at a time when I pushed my walker along the ground, and no longer improved, despite the use only of my left hand. For that matter, my whole arm was no better either. I was ready at my next appointment with Dr. Whitney with my biggest worry of all.

Maybe I could see the world about me, but I didn't feel alive in it. Very gradually, I realized, my mind missed something. I understood who and where I was, but I didn't *feel* them at all. Things were no more real to me than they were in my comascape, in some ways considerably less so, because the places and experiences in my coma fully satisfied all my senses.

"It's the difference between *perceived* and *emotional* truth," I pleaded. "I don't feel *connected*."

Instead of some advice as to what to do about it, Dr. Whitney noted my phrase down carefully in the chart. As I watched him scribble my words, I started to wonder just how much my doctors knew and, during many rest periods back on the cot, to ask myself how many other open questions there might be.

A second visit to the orthopedic surgeon disheartened me more, because Dr. Brien seemed so satisfied with my progress. He stood in front of the illuminated X-rays that showed the titanium implants in my pelvis as white cutouts over the milky curves of my bones, and radiated the optimism of a job well done.

"When do I next see you?" I asked.

"Oh, come back in the next eight to nine months."

An eye specialist was no more helpful. I was afflicted by a periodic red eye—"Dracula eye," I called it, because it went that red. The doctor checked to make sure my retina wasn't scratched, and in subsequent visits prescribed antibiotic drops of increasing potency, as Dracula eye obstinately recurred. And no one could tell me what I needed to know most: how to plug in my heart and soul, to make the world I saw feel real.

I had the recommendation from my Intensive Care nurses to see Dr. Alan Brodney, who was an expert in a specialty I'd not heard of, "developmental optometry." His offices were on the Westside, and I liked Alan immediately. Judy and Marilyn on the front desk were energized and enthusiastic too, all committed to vision as a process that could be rehabilitated.

It would have been difficult not to like them. It turned out Alan was in the audience of *Howie from Maui*, an HBO live concert special I produced with Howie Mandel. By coincidence, he was on vacation at Waikiki Beach with friends from optometry school, came to the show, and watched me onstage in a repeating cameo appearance, in black leather shoes and grass skirt. Now my vision depended on him.

The examination optometrists generally give to check an adult for eyeglasses seemed insignificant compared to Dr. Brodney's investigation. When he was done, he told my mother that almost nothing remained of my left peripheral vision. He didn't know how much of it he could revive, but agreed to try.

There would be all kinds of visual exercises in his office, three times a week.

There were stereo viewfinders, a rotating wheel with patterns to watch, and a biofeedback machine to improve vision, just on that first day. Brodney sent me home with some optical illusions on cards. A stairway that changed before my eyes between a view from above and from below, depending on how you looked at it; another card could be a black goblet, or two white faces in profile; another, a set of white arrows that pointed up, or black ones that pointed sideways. My task with each was to gain control of my vision, make my brain see either alternative at will. The challenge exhausted and exhilarated me because, just maybe, Dr. Brodney could help me reconnect with the world.

The business of caring pressured my mother all the time. While unpaid hospital bills piled up, Pauline Rossi called and grilled my mother about whether or not I showed steady improvement, a stress that lasted until whoever was senior to her said "yes," Great-West paid, and the next review began. But the bigger problem was how to justify Cedars outpatient therapy when I received only one session every few days. The pressure was heaviest on my mother who ferried me there, an hour-and-a-half round trip for forty-five minutes of care. One afternoon, she dropped me off for another monthly visit with Dr. Whitney, and left to do errands. Whitney wasn't there, so I waited in his office, and gazed out the window.

It was a nice spring day, and I liked the way the cars shone, as they drove by in the street below. I still liked them when my mother returned an hour later.

"Where's Whitney?" she demanded.

"I don't know," was my placid reply.

It hadn't occurred to me the length of the wait made a difference, disabled long enough to forget that I could influence the outside world, instead of simply look at it through a window.

She stormed off to find him, while his secretary escorted me to the elevator. I stood there, unsteadily propped on my walker, and heard their argument continue as they approached.

"Why are you so upset?" Dr. Whitney asked. "The patient isn't."

"Of course he's not upset," my mother retorted angrily. "If Simon was normal he'd be angry, but he's *not*. He barely knows he's here!"

Dr. Whitney decided to shift gears; that is, make it her problem.

"Maybe you should come in and discuss your feelings, and that might help you cope?" he reasoned.

In truth, her anger was in part due to his refusal to apologize for his failure to show up, but also her certainty that my recovery was stalled. Cedars, one of the biggest and best hospitals in L.A., didn't seem able to help me, and it was ever harder for my mother to convince herself, let alone Pauline Rossi, that the expense was justified. My discharge from Cedars looked not so much like a stepping-stone to the next level of recovery, but the end of it. Pauline was a nurse, but made no suggestions of alternatives, any facility other than Cedars, or that there might be a better place for me to go for treatment, and of course neither did Cedars. No one tells you everything you need to know to find and follow the hidden path to full recovery.

My mother could cope. Like my father, she'd lived through a World War and was very resilient. But when she asked herself the logical, practical question—what more could be done to save me—she faced the possibility that my situation was hopeless; that there was nothing more she or my father could do. She felt despondent, and she felt helpless. Until she had an idea.

CHAPTER ELEVEN

FASTER, HARDER, BETTER

Once in a while you get shown the light
In the strangest of places if you look at it right
                    —The Grateful Dead,
                        "Scarlet Begonias"

My mother was at her local Target store, worried even there about what to do next. She assumed all hospitals were about the same, so it was hopeless if Cedars couldn't help. She stopped suddenly, amongst the merchandise, when it struck her: this Target was near another hospital. On her way home, on impulse, she pulled into the parking lot of Northridge Hospital. Nobody drops into a hospital. It's not that sort of place, and she didn't know what to expect, at her wits' end as she approached the front desk.

"My son's been at Cedars for five months, and I don't know what to do," was all she could say, and then told the receptionist the tragic story.

"We have a special head injury rehab program," offered Debbie Flaherty, the director of rehab services, when paged to the reception. "Would you like to see it?"

She saw the answer in my mother's eyes, and called on her cell.

My first sign of change was a gentle hint by my parents, about "a house" where I would stay. It's often difficult for head injury patients to cope with change, and I was scared. Patricia Klein, the program coordinator, came to our home herself, to assess my suitability. A kind woman, she told us about TGIC, the special outpatient program Northridge Hospital offered. The initials stood for "Thank God I Care", and it provided intensive rehabilitation every weekday, dedicated to stroke and brain-injured patients. After her interview, Patricia said she'd recommend a full evaluation.

It was hard to grasp that one of the best rehab programs in the United States was less than seven miles from my home, yet during five months at Cedars no one there so much as hinted the place existed. If not for my mother's moment of inspiration that day at Target, my recovery would have ended shortly at Cedars. Almost a million Americans survive strokes each year, many to find their ability to walk, talk, or work compromised; that they are dependent on others for the most basic tasks. After limited therapy, insurance typically then provides a wheelchair or cane, leaves patients to manage as best they can, and their recovery stops.

My mother's inspiration saved me from this fate, and shone a light on the reality that recovery isn't only a choice patients must make; it's a quest they must undertake if they want to find the hidden path. Great-West's written confirmation arrived the day before I was due to enroll, and that very next morning I was on my way, with wheelchair, walker, and insurance card, as nervous as a boy on his first day of school. As I stared

out the car, I wondered what "nice home" we were headed toward.

I remembered the show jackets I once ordered for
a crew at the start of principal photography. "Age Old
Friends" announced the title of my movie about an old
age home across the back, and I wrote a motto for the
front: "faster, harder, better." It was my exhortation to
the crew of how we would work to make our film special,
but felt as though it was the motto for my therapists
at Cedars. I had deeply mixed feelings about the ever
more optimistic and unrealistic goals they set in my
short sessions.

It began to dawn on me that the pace of recovery
was set by outside forces. Great-West's approval was
for me to attend only three days for intensive tests. I'd
no idea what they were, what was to become of me if I
failed the evaluation, or the consequences if I fell behind this accelerated and artificial pace. All I knew that
morning was that, like most all my injuries, my gradual
improvement at Cedars was a lot slower than the therapists needed. Would my final recovery leave me as a living dead—a zombie with a dead brain? Panic turned to
dread as we approached Northridge Hospital.

There was a small, one-story house on the other
side of Etiwanda Avenue from the main hospital, the
kind you'd never notice unless you looked for it. From
the curb, a carefully maintained pathway led across a
manicured lawn, to a small ramp to a freshly painted
front door.

As my mother rolled my wheelchair toward it,
an African-American woman, who beamed the biggest
smile of welcome, opened the door.

"Hi! I'm Ola!" she called, and explained as we approached how she'd watched out for our arrival through
the front window, how I was in great hands now, and
how my mother should return to pick me up at five.

Once inside, Ola showed me around the TGIC facility that was specifically designed to provide rehabilitative healthcare, rather than general medical and surgical services like Cedars.

The house hadn't changed much since its donation to the hospital. Off the lobby was a kitchen, living room, and a short hallway, formerly to bedrooms, now rooms equipped for therapy and offices, including Patricia Klein's. Some simple exercise equipment was installed in the garage, for physical therapy.

"Anything more complicated and we use the hospital—like we use their bus for outings," Ola explained.

She brought me back to the entrance lobby where Patricia came out of her office to join us. I explained how, at Cedars, I got two therapy sessions twice a week.

"I'll show you what we do *here*," Patricia said, and pointed to a notice board on the wall.

At the start of the short hallway off the lobby, was a schedule for each of their patients. "At TGIC we call them 'clients,'" Patricia offered.

"Depending on your evaluation, Simon, your name would be up there," she added, and explained that assessment of my potential for recovery would take at least the three days that were authorized.

It was too hard to read and listen at the same time, so I scarcely heard Patricia as I scanned the sheet of paper. My limited vision slowly understood the top row was a workweek of Monday through Friday. Then it occurred to my brain, as an entirely unconnected step, to read the left column, which yielded hours of the day from nine to five with a gap for lunch. Patricia realized my difficulty and used her finger to trace across each weekday, a model of continuous care with therapies in physical, occupational, community/recreational, cognitive, neuro-psychology, speech, and more. It was perfect if, I silently prayed, I could pass the evaluation.

Patricia introduced me to Jean Markarian, a speech pathologist who'd supervise it.

"Green Jean was my nickname when I grew up," she began. "Know why?"

Jean was a very attractive Californian with bright blue eyes. As she planned, she drew my attention to them, while I pondered why anyone would call her that.

"Because I swam all the time in high school, and the chlorine used to make my blonde hair turn green," Jean laughed.

Five minutes later, after she distracted my mind with forms to complete and other tasks, she tested me. "Do you remember my nickname, and how I got it?" she quizzed.

I desperately wished I could, that my mind could pay closer attention to what it was told. I felt such intense pressure to pass this, my first test. I knew Jean's interesting personal story was something a normal person would remember for a while, but it had slid far down the slope of my thoughts.

I struggled to draw it back up into the light, while Jean patiently waited to see if my damaged brain could retrieve the information, and I felt infinite gratitude when it finally surfaced, and I could repeat the story.

There would, Jean explained to my parents at the end of that first day, be monthly evaluations contributed to by each therapist at TGIC to build a complete analysis of me.

As TGIC continued its evaluation, I came to know the therapists, and confided my fear of failure to one, Beryl, as she methodically tested my muscles in the garage-turned-gym.

"Don't worry, Simon," she assured me, as she worked with what looked like a super-sized compass from a high school geometry class, to measure how far my arm could move in its range of motion. When TGIC's report arrived, it was hard to remember that the person the group described in such detail was me. I felt an odd sense of disassociation, as if someone else, who happened to share the name Simon Lewis, was under consideration for treatment. The evaluation covered everything from issues of laundry and clothing care, to home and financial management. It included a discussion of my ideas to return to productive activity, and barriers to it. I explained my career as producer and adjunct professor at USC to Jean; how my family kept in touch with the dean there, but with no idea when I could do anything.

Unlike the limited evaluations at Cedars—and in my favor—TGIC's multipage analysis noted that "strengths include: strong desire to return to some form of productive activity, insight into deficits, and good interpersonal skills." Five months after the crash, TGIC determined I was eligible for rehab and, with goals established, ready to enter its therapy program.

My first Monday morning began in the living room with a group session led by Dr. Sally Turner, a thoughtful and dynamic African-American physician. She introduced herself as the team's neuropsychologist to the other fresh clients whose names I saw on the timetable, my first new people in so long who weren't medics.

Ted introduced himself first, an air traffic controller who had an aneurysm—a ruptured blood vessel in his brain—without warning one day at work. And then Pete, a builder who fell from a ladder and hit his head; Carol, whose life was changed one day when a rock, dropped from an overpass by vandals, crashed through her windshield; and Chris, who was quite distinctive because he wore a cyclist's helmet, on doctor's orders, to protect his skull while it strengthened. Chris explained in his introduction to the group how he ran the stage lights for a community college theatre until one day, he saw a new school employee give him a strange look. It was nearly the last thought Chris ever had, because the new employee took a hammer to Chris's head.

There was Zack, a young construction worker and biker. Like Chris, he remembered few details, but was told afterwards that he was clipped by a truck, came off his Harley, and flew twenty feet before his head hit a wall. I liked Zack. As he listened to Chris tell his story, Zack reacted straight from his heart.

"Man . . . ," he sympathized, "that's really fucked!"

One possible result of head injury is a loss of self-control, called lability, revealed by coarse language, neglect of personal appearance, and a general disregard for conventional rules of social conduct. So there was a medical reason why Sally politely remonstrated.

"Now do you think that's an appropriate thing to say, Zack?"

"Huh?" he wondered aloud, then fell silent while he considered what to say to this attractive young woman, who was his doctor. I understood Zack's language might not be appropriate and wondered if maybe I suffered from lability too, because it didn't seem to matter if Zack used those words. What mattered was he came through his injury with mental capacity to form a thought and express it. And the other thing, it seemed to me, was how right Zack was, about what had happened to us all. I tried to focus.

"Now that we're introduced," Sally said, "we're going to spend this hour on assertiveness training."

This aspect of my injuries was never so much as broached by therapists at Cedars, but in this session I discovered how badly I needed counseling. In my own introduction to the group, I described the hit-and-run, but not how I was married, and that my wife had died.

I knew I'd be unable to continue if I tried talking about her, and was grateful my schedule for the week included a private session with Sally. The group pressed on with training, as our doctor described how damage to the brain often weakened both initiation and assertiveness, made us each like a child who does what it's told—which we must learn to overcome.

"You have choices, can always choose to say no," Sally offered, and then began to tell us the "rescuer and victim" paradox.

"Imagine there's a drowning man in a river who's helpless. 'Save me!' he cries to a passerby. . . ."

Sally was a good storyteller, and had everyone's attention.

"Now, the passerby—the rescuer—feels flattered," Sally explained, "because we all like to help people. It makes us feel good. We're proud to play an important role, to save someone who's in trouble."

She had that right. I remembered how good it felt to help others in need.

"So the rescuer helps the victim out of the river," Sally continued, "and goes home, and so does the victim. All live happily ever after in the parable."

We listened to her nice story. I especially liked the happy ending, where TGIC came to our rescue.

"But in the real world," Sally continued, "what tends to happen is that someone isn't actually about to drown; they just *think* so, *think* they're helpless. And in real life, there are *no rescuers*."

From the uneasy glances, I could see everyone in the group shared the same thought: if there were no rescuers, what chance did we have?

"Oh, a passerby will help you to some extent," Sally answered our unspoken doubts. "To the extent of help they feel comfortable to offer. But in the real world, they don't have the resources to save you. So the help is ultimately insufficient."

Sally headed to the point she needed her group of trauma patients to understand.

"In real life," she looked at us with deep care, "patients who allow themselves to play the role of victims, who wait for a rescuer to come along, tend to live unhappily ever after."

It was a sobering thought.

"There are no rescuers," Sally concluded. "But you are not helpless."

For the rest of the hour, we participated in some role-playing games, and practiced how to politely refuse invitations, instead of agreeing to everything we were asked to do. For the first time, I had another therapy directly after, and Patricia arranged that I could simply stay in the living room armchair and nap for twenty minutes to prepare. TGIC was a fantastic, flexible program. Next up, I met with Jean in her small room, one of the converted bedrooms off the hallway. She began with some word puzzles.

"There are seven planets in the 'ss,'" she said.

"Solar system?" seemed to float out of my mind. There were a bunch more, a few of which I got. Next, she tried me on a very simple computer game. There was text on the computer screen, but no pictures. The idea was to see if I could imagine the world the text described, and draw it. It was a child's game, to gather clues, and make a map to find some hidden treasure.

"You have come to a big rock in a field," announced the monitor.

"Turn left," I pecked out with my good right forefinger on the keyboard. Nothing.

Hmmm.

"Turn right," I tried.

No good either. The only other direction I could think of was "turn back" and I knew that was wrong. I was stumped.

"What if there's something *on top* of the rock?" Jean tried.

I drew a mental blank. My therapist waited, to see if I could figure out how to find the next clue without another prompt, but I was stuck.

"What if you climb *up* the rock?" she finally suggested.

Disabled so long, unable to climb even one step, I'd forgotten it was possible. "Up" no longer existed in my mind as a direction for my body to go. Sure enough, the clue was on top of the rock; a graphic demonstration of the climb ahead for my mind as well, to cope with the simplest of life's questions.

The next day was the outing in the Northridge Hospital bus described by Ola when I arrived, something Cedars wasn't equipped to provide. Some clients had to plan the trip, and learn again how to read a Los Angeles road map, grasp the spatial relationships on it, make choices of the best route, and write out their directions clearly enough for other clients to read them, and call out directions in the bus.

It was rehabilitation of the most helpful kind: goal-oriented therapy to develop effective living skills. Pete and Ted selected and planned this outing. Ola, ever patient and encouraging, drove. Chris, in his helmet, and I rode shotgun, and peered every which way but the right one through the windshield, as we tried to follow Zack and Carol's written and verbal directions. We were headed to a program for the disabled called Access to Sailing, run by a wheelchair-bound captain. The plan was to go out on his boat and sail in Long Beach Harbor—if we made it.

"South on the 405," Zack the biker called out from the back once again.

"Which lane do I take for the 405 *south*?" Ola insisted for a third time.

She still sounded cheerful, but this time there was unmistakable urgency in her voice.

"Come on, guys, make up your mind!" Pete pleaded, while Ted stayed silent.

Chris and I had both lost some vision from our strokes. We had that in common, too. We looked at the row of signs across the freeway, tried to grasp which sign belonged to which lane as the interchange approached fast. We debated the point, but couldn't decide between the two of us as time began to run out. The intersection looked huge and bewildering, and it was hard to believe I ever made these choices with ease.

"One . . . two . . . three. . . . How about the fourth?" Chris tried.

"Looks good to me!" I nodded, and thought even now, with Ola behind the wheel, how nervous I was to commit to what my eyes saw.

"Glad you guys finally decided!" Ola laughed, as she neatly executed a double lane change at the last second.

Once out in the harbor, the blue beauty of the ocean, its gentle movement under our boat, comforted me. That, and the sight of the seals that sunned themselves on an ocean buoy, barking and twitching their whiskers at us as we came close. Ashore, we went into a restaurant for lunch, my first in regular clothes. It was key to TGIC's rehabilitation program to challenge every client's deficits; it was hard and embarrassing to move between the tables with my walker and for my new friends, it was hard to function in the outside world for different reasons: how to read a menu when your vision is limited; to remember what it is you like to eat, and make the decision to order it; how to use a credit card to pay; or to remember there is something called rush-hour traffic, and to plan ahead what time to leave.

As the week advanced, I got to know other TGIC therapists, and had my first private session with Sally. She explained that the other therapists knew my case history, and wouldn't discuss Marcy unless I felt comfortable with that.

She began on the safe ground of childhood, and asked if I remembered my first book. It was, I managed to recall, a fantasy adventure called *The Weirdstone of Brisingamen*, that takes its readers to the same world as *Harry Potter* and *Lord of the Rings*, a world of mystery and fantasy that's within our own, if you know how to step sideways into it. The image that stayed with me was of a cavern filled with knights in shining armor, protected by a magic light. The knights rested under a spell, ready when called to ride forth and rescue our world. I told Sally maybe that was how I felt about all life, that it was precious, and we had hidden resources, noble knights within, reserves of strength ready to protect us in our hour of need.

Sally brought me to when I was ten and began to make films, then a fourteen-year-old who wanted to make the most of each day.

"I don't know the job I want, but it's not nine to five," I explained to an oil executive on school career day. Told to prepare a five-minute speech on my goals, that's all I came up with on what I wanted of the future: to make all of it count. My interviewer got very animated.

"You come see me next year, and I'll take you places. You'll see oil fields round the clock, round the globe," he rapid-fired back.

As it turned out, my family hatched our plan to move to America after dinner one evening, I explained to Sally. To fit in Cambridge, I applied early and was accepted.

In my last year there, the fact that my family

was in Los Angeles persuaded Christ's College to let me share a big house normally reserved for visiting professors with my buddy Mike. On graduation day, I gave him the keys to my car that I bought with summer jobs, my stereo system already loaded into it.

"Have fun with them, Mike. I'm out of here!" I grinned.

He looked a bit stunned by the gifts, but they were of use to him and no longer to me, so I thought it made perfect sense.

"Simon," he pondered, "I've had this whole year to observe you quite closely. . . ." My friend the history graduate paused to consider the fruits gained from his yearlong study. "And I've just realized something," he said thoughtfully. "Under your completely rational exterior, you are, in fact . . . completely crazy!"

We shared a final laugh and headed for the ceremony. My parents had joined me for graduation, and the next day, we flew together to join my brothers in Los Angeles.

My psychotherapist listened to and encouraged me as I pieced together happy memories, but her next questions brought me back to the arena of blank despair I felt at Cedars; how I felt I lived in a silent landscape, like Narcissus, who gazed for eternity into a pool of water, except I didn't want to see myself; how I sat by my pool and gazed into the reflection of Marcy's memory, and how I felt closest to her when there were no ripples to disturb it, felt closest when I was silent about her.

Sally listened, as I asked her if it was okay that I still cried a lot at night. How at those times I felt, by my pool, as if I could hear a waterfall behind me; that I could turn and dimly see Marcy directly through the waterfall, but never move through it to her; how the waterfall that separated us was made of tears, hers and mine. And Sally assured it was okay, how each of us grieves in our own way.

As summer advanced, there were more outings, some with bittersweet memories. We went to The Huntington in Pasadena, where months earlier Marcy was the event planner for a Music Center fundraiser. In August, I was taken to the Department of Motor Vehicles and shown how to get in line for a California photo ID, to replace my vanished driver's license. There are points in your life when you need a reason to smile for the camera and at that frozen moment in time, it was beyond me; it took all of my concentration to stand there upright.

More therapists, with different specialties, were added as my mother ferried me back and forth, one called Emily included, for it was she who walked me fifty yards to the special pool inside Northridge Hospital for regular aquatic therapy. Although I depended on Emily's assistance, I knew that every step took me closer to my first goal at Cedars. Fifty yards to the pool and back meant that I finally walked a hundred yards in the outside world.

There was an extra joy, of how good the water felt both physically and mentally, when Emily expertly moved me down the wide shallow steps, specially designed for disabled access, into the Northridge Hospital therapy pool.

Once in the water, the struggle it took to get there vanished as Emily suspended me in the extra warm, womb-like water with my flotation device and water wings, and asked me to move my arms and legs. Before we left the hospital, she started me in a pottery and crafts group there, to continue to test and rebuild fine motor skills in my hands and fingers.

TGIC cost $535 per day; so much less than the cost of Cedars, you might think it would make things easier. My family certainly thought it would, as I benefited from the far more intensive program and graduated from walker to quad cane to single-point cane.

But suddenly, it got harder to obtain approval, and demand calls came from Northridge Hospital for payment. All too soon, my parents were forced to tell me I was cut from five days a week of therapy to four. When Pauline Rossi called to say that, based on TGIC's progress reports, she recommended I be cut to three days—and soon thereafter terminate recovery at TGIC—my mother snapped.

"You sit up in Denver making decisions about what's best for my son? You come down here and see what TGIC is doing. They're *wonderful*."

"Yes," Pauline answered, calm and unswayed, "that's why I think Simon's ready to move on. Do all his therapy at home."

"They're trying to save my son's life and you're killing him!" my mother cried down the phone. "Who can I speak to?" she began to shout. "I *have* to talk to someone higher up."

Her vigilance, her readiness to fight for my care, again kept me on the hidden path. When Pauline transferred my swollen file to end the call, we came to deal directly with Great-West's Catastrophic Claims Division, staffed by individuals who themselves faced long-term health issues. Under their direct oversight, Great-West readily evaluated medical complications, which cropped up frequently. At my annual checkup, I consulted my regular internist Dr. Terrill about one. It was Terrill who spotted my critical white cell count from gangrene when my family urgently called him into Cedars, so I trusted him totally. I pointed to one area of pain.

"What's this lumpy area that hurts?"

"That's your pelvis," came his answer.

Nor could he answer why my Dracula red eye flared repeatedly, and my debilitating fatigue didn't improve. TGIC's monthly reports described this barrier to recovery, but offered no ideas either as to the cause or a solution, so I went to see Bruce Kern, the neurosurgeon who opened my head, saved my life, and installed plates in my skull to hold it together, for answers

It was October 10, my first wedding anniversary, I reflected numbly as I waited to see him. I forced my mind to turn away, before it could dwell on how many couples celebrate their first anniversary with the sound of a new voice in the world, and the silence in my life now. Forced it back to this one moment, and the next step of recovery.

It was strange to meet this eminent neurosurgeon for the second time with no recollection of the first. A serious and quiet man, Dr. Kern explained what he did to save my life at that encounter, on his operating table the night of the crash.

He used a model skull to demonstrate where he installed the metal plates in my head, and how he was forced to wait for the results of the emergency aortogram before he could operate.

"That wait's another reason your brain injury is so massive," he concluded.

Dr. Kern was done, but I wasn't. I desperately needed this expert's help to diagnose and explain my constant fatigue, the sense of a constant pressure that weighed down my thoughts, so I could understand what happened inside my brain during my every waking moment.

"Doctor, I feel like there's this elephant . . . and it's sitting on my head. Do you think it would help if you took out the titanium?"

"No," he assured with finality. In his professional opinion, the head hardware was not an issue and should remain in my skull for the rest of my life. He recommended I visit a brain-mapping program at a downtown clinic. Its conclusions, such as "reflexes: 3+ on the left,

left Babinski: right toe downgoing," provided no helpful answers to what I could do about something called
"Babinski."

I fared similarly with Dr. Birnbaum, my dentist
of many years who I trusted to treat my jaw injury. One
thing that so completely hides the path to full recovery
is that unless you ask the right questions at the right
time, no one tells you everything you need to know.
When I visited Dr. Birnbaum for the first time since
the crash, there was an infection, or fistula, in my jaw.
Perhaps my fatigue was a result of the infection, so he
sent me to an endodontist to remove it.

Two root canals later, the infection remained. It
was the first time I realized that the doctors I depended
on before the crash to keep me healthy might make mistakes. Because it was only then that it occurred to me
to ask a really obvious question, as I looked up from the
chair.

"How many . . . root canalshh . . . you plan . . . find
. . . infection?" I mumbled to the oral surgeon.

And I saw from the look on his face that he didn't
know.

Like most stroke and trauma victims, I confronted what looked like the premature end of recovery; the
sinking feeling that I was nearly "done" as far as my
doctors could tell. That in spite of my debilitating symptoms, there was little more they could do to diagnose
and cure them, and no hint of a way forward.

In December, there was a Christmas party at
TGIC, complete with a tree and refreshments, therapists and clients, all new friends. The outing that week
was to a local Bloomingdale's, my first trip to a department store since the accident, to hear the music, gaze at
the twinkling Christmas decorations, and see the world
move on with nothing changed—which simultaneously
comforted and disconcerted me. This year of my life was

near an end.

I came to an escalator and paused, not sure how to step on safely. How fast the handrail moved! I felt a weird disassociation as I looked down. I could see patterns the fluorescent lights made on the steel fins, where they appeared from under the floor to create that moving first step. They seemed to dance in time to the Christmas carols over the store speakers. I looked up at the perennially familiar, suddenly banal store merchandise, and all the holiday decorations and special sales that surrounded me.

It was so strange to experience death, then return to see the world go on the same. I felt a deep continuation of one of my earliest memories at Cedars, that I was an observer from another planet with no links to this space or time. I looked again at the aluminum steps go round and round, so much faster than I could walk. Going nowhere. I didn't know if my recovery could make any more real progress than those steps, if the business of caring was set to cut off therapy before doctors could even stop my jaw infection. And I remembered that Peggy Lee song again.

Is that all there is . . . to my recovery?

"Maybe this is my plateau?" I mumbled to myself, as I finally began my first escalator ride.

Though he put me into shock the last time he treated me, I returned to Cedars to see Dr. Anderson. I felt bonded with the team who saved my life—and Anderson looked like my last chance to find the answers for my broken jaw that eluded my dentist.

It made me smile to see him again, but not for long. Never one to delay, he examined the infection, and then thoroughly cauterized it. I felt flesh burn deep, as he scoured both infection and living tissue from my jaw, and doubted whether I'd done the right thing.

I doubted it more when I returned next week,

because the mystery infection remained, invulnerable. Only then did he ask,

"Simon, did we ever get a panorex of you?"

It was, he clarified, an X-ray that tracks around the jaw and shows the whole mandible. When he pulled my hospital chart, the answer, frustratingly, was no. By the time that I could be moved, my jaw was wired, and no one thought to do one since.

With Dr. Anderson's prescription in hand, it cost a mere sixty dollars at a storefront clinic to get one taken, and we were back next day for him to put the image up on his light panel.

"Oh! You have osteomyelitis," he said simply.

The hardware he installed, and my jaw along with it, was infected. It's not unusual in cases of major trauma, as blood and body fluids mix with the outside world. It might be nice if someone warned you, but doctors don't mention possibilities until a symptom requires diagnosis. Which means that if you're not vigilant, problems can remain undiagnosed, your potential to achieve full recovery stalled, until it's too late.

It was December 28. Two days later, I checked into Cedars for tests, for Dr. Phil Anderson to operate on me again January 3, and to begin my first New Year at Cedars.

CHAPTER TWELVE

MEET DOCTOR FEELGOOD

One pill makes you larger
And one pill makes you small
Go ask Alice
When she's ten feet tall
                    —Jefferson Airplane,
                        "White Rabbit"

The life-threatening diagnosis explained my recovery plateau, and required immediate surgery to remove the hardware and scrape out all infected bone. I was temporarily discharged from TGIC, and on my first conscious trip to Cedars for scheduled surgery, fear became terror as a nurse did her blood work, attached a baggage tag to my wrist, and rolled me off to meet my first anesthesiologist. "Doctor Feelgood," as I'd come to name every practitioner who put me under for surgery, after a mind-numbing heavy rock band, whose concerts I enjoyed in my days as a Cambridge student.

"How much do you weigh, Mr. Lewis?" he innocently asked, as he looked in my eyes and smiled—a
successful ploy to distract me, then slipped in my IV.

As I answered him, sure enough, he made me *feel
goood*. I'd no worries at all; I couldn't even remember
what one felt like.

In his operation, Dr. Anderson found deep infection, and in a procedure called a debridement, reported
his removal of both it and the titanium hardware. Maybe it was Doctor Feelgood's drugs that gave me a rush
of focus, or perhaps the adrenaline surge of antibiotics
that flooded through my system, but as I lay in my room
after surgery, I knew it was time to make some kind of
decision, if I only knew what it was.

I asked to see the hardware Anderson removed,
and stared at the little bag of titanium pieces, bright
and shiny in the morning light. I puzzled what decision
my mind knew had to be made, that I couldn't retrieve.
I wondered why, if Anderson found the cause both of my
fatigue and bouts of Dracula eye, I didn't feel better now
that it was gone and I was disease free.

With the rest of America, I was distracted when
the New Year also brought the start of the trial of that
decade, of O.J. Simpson. I felt so disassociated from the
world, but connected instantly with this crime. When
we first met, my wife and her roommates lived yards
from the murder scene in an identical building. I walked
along the same side alley countless times to visit Marcy,
and recognized the layout, knew how trapped those two
victims were.

After my discharge from Cedars, my mind inescapably returned to the nagging decision that somehow
related to my future, and the bag of metal parts, which
for some reason I brought home with me. Perhaps in-
tuitively, far down the slope of consciousness, my brain
urged my attention. But high on the slope, the only

conscious thought to break through was a question: whether I should keep the other hardware in my body. When I asked nurses and doctors for advice they smiled, shrugged, and told me not to worry about it, "unless you have pain."

All I knew for sure was that they never warned me about this major hardware problem because they *hadn't known*. And as I wondered what else my doctors might not know, an answer dawned on me: to take the hardware out. Great-West had already reduced my days at TGIC, and this solved what would happen if doctors found a problem after the carrier closed my claim. It must all come out while I had insurance, not wait for a doctor's recommendation.

All of us wonder if we're in the right medical hands; worry about it even as the business of caring progressively limits our choice of doctors—and makes it ever more critical to figure out. With limited knowledge, I tried to reconsider Dr. Anderson, who helped save me and protected my hearing, but tore out my wires without anesthetic. And there remained the question of why he hadn't done a panorex earlier.

As the year advanced, my doubts crept across to my dependable dentist with the comforting smile, who ordered two root canals before I canceled any more shots in the dark. I liked my idea when I returned to TGIC, because the pace stepped up. Their physiatrist—a physician specialized in physical medicine and rehabilitation—recommended I wear an AFO, a rigid brace "to be used with improving efficiency for longer distances and fast-paced gait," except I didn't want a fix to walk faster. What I needed, desperately, was to walk *better*.

"Why does my pelvis still hurt?" I asked Dr. Avidan. "Is it possible that's why I can't walk?"

She didn't know. If my medical team missed a life-threatening disease like osteomyelitis, which of them could give me an answer I could trust? I wondered again when I returned to Dr. Birnbaum in the fall, for yet more dental X-rays.

"Good news!" he said with a smile. "The fistula's closing . . . and all's well!"

That was when I lost confidence in him. After the root canals, cauterization, and debridement, the fistula infection was "closing"—not closed. When my eyes again turned blood red and I inspected my latest Dracula eye in the mirror, I felt something was wrong with the hardware inside my body, but with no clue where to turn or who to ask for advice. The answer was literally next door.

Our neighbor Harry, a network news producer for ABC, previously lived next door to an orthopedic surgeon at Cedars. Whereas Dr. Brien skillfully installed my hardware, Harry told my parents that Dr. Robert Klapper was a surgeon who specialized in its removal. As with my mother's discovery of TGIC, we learned about this medical option through pure luck. With Harry's information, we were well prepared when I attended my follow-up with Dr. Brien, to assess the pain in my pelvis that radiated down my left leg.

There was the same unmistakably cool tone in his clinic, that this talented surgeon who rebuilt my body with titanium didn't want or need to see me. Brien checked his incisions and the radiology images, as I explained my need to remove his titanium implants.

"I'll remove the back pelvis hardware if you want, to help your pain," he evaluated, "but not the front—it was a hard enough job to put it in."

That same day, we drove on to Dr. Klapper. It was the first time I sought a second opinion, and had no idea whether it was realistic to think a different surgeon would reach another conclusion, or if it was wise to question the advice of a doctor who opened my body, saw all, and showed the courage and skill to save me.

But his clinic seemed impressive. There was a friendly and beautiful receptionist, Bibi, and a very professional assistant in his thirties.

"Hi, I'm Mark!" he introduced himself brightly, shortly after I completed the patient questionnaire. "As in, *mark* my words," he added slowly.

He'd reviewed my questionnaire, knew of my head injury, and wanted to help me remember his name. This was a kind and caring place, I thought, even if I then waited an eternity in the reception. To pass the time, I gazed at an aquarium filled with exotic tropical fish, which gazed blankly back. There was also time to study a life-size picture of Wilt Chamberlain, the pro basketball legend. Wilt stood next to—more like towered above—another man, his orthopedic surgeon Dr. Klapper. It was another clue I was in the right place, which is that you can partly assess a doctor by the quality of the staff and clientele they attract and keep.

Finally, I was led into a cubicle where Robert arrived. Cheerful, energized, and almost bouncy, he chatted about Harry, our mutual neighbor, and checked the images I brought.

"Yes, your pelvis looks okay—but I can remove the back hardware if it's causing problems."

It was half what I hoped, and not so different than Dr. Brien's medical advice. At least Robert sounded enthusiastic it might help.

"What about the *front* of my pelvis?" I tried.

I showed him the painful lump my internist Dr. Terrill examined and told me was "just my pelvis." Robert shook his head.

"No, that's not your pelvis—it's your titanium plate. To try and get that thing out is what we call a long run for a short slide. Don't recommend it. Let's book you for surgery on the back!"

While I waited, the state of California passed my case over to Federal Social Security, and called me in for an interview.

When the government's doctor asked about my plans for the future, I couldn't see past my next encounter with Doctor Feelgood, and felt torn between the short-term view imposed by the risks of my next surgery, and the long view that recovery takes. On the one hand, I was expected by Social Security to return to work; on the other, doctors were about to draw pints of my blood for an emergency transfusion if something went wrong, reminding me of just how short my future might be. In fact, David Roy, a writer-director and old friend, had asked me to produce his first film. Out of a desire to help, I met with the financier, my first attempt to put a movie deal together and, for that matter, my first business encounter of any kind. But I wasn't able to cope, the mental overload instant, which forced me to withdraw from the project. When their decision arrived, Social Security's three-year approval of me for federal disability came as a relief, but I began to wonder if that would be long enough, and to worry what would happen to me if it wasn't.

Emily, my recreational therapist, got me into the hospital pool every week for aquatic therapy, and though her reports noted that my swimming skills "remain non-functional at this time," her sessions helped in more subtle ways.

As my mind reached out repeatedly to my nearly weightless body, in one session it occurred to me that if no one could tell me how to help my brain heal, I'd try to rebuild it from remembered components of my old life.

Toward the end of that session, Emily set down a very small box for me to step onto, a child's step, on the floor of the pool. I strained with every atom of my being to find my body parts, to spark the response I needed from each nerve pathway in the correct sequence. To lift my knee for that box was just like a step over a small fence, so I imagined one in front of me; looked within to find a sense memory of the whole.

And, heavily propped against Emily in the pool, my mind found the whole of my weightless body, my leg lifted . . . and I stepped up.

March 3, two years and a day after the crash, came for Dr. Klapper to take out the thirteen screws and two plates from the back of my pelvis, for the "radical resection with removal foreign body deep."

"The risks and complications are great," the surgery report began, followed by the mantra used by surgeons, that you can always get better, always die, on the operating table.

I survived, and watched the O.J. Simpson saga continue as I recuperated in my room. I remembered I was a California attorney, and tried to keep up with the lawyers as I drifted in and out of consciousness.

I was discharged home too soon, because the wound reopened and I was rushed to Dr. Klapper's clinic. It felt great to see him so cheerful. It's always good to see your surgeon smile after a surgery.

"You must have been in terrible pain whenever you sat down," he said as he disinfected and restapled another ten-inch scar line.

"There were these long calcium spikes, Simon, that grew on the screw heads—to right up under your skin!"

He held his thumb and forefinger apart by over an inch to demonstrate just how long the undetected bone spikes were.

"There was bone mass all around the plates too," he added, and dropped them, now clean and shiny, into my collection bag to join the jaw hardware.

These were huge lumps of metal by comparison,

and I was so grateful plates, screws, spikes, and all, were no longer inside me. I wondered why I felt no pain, why no one could tell me before, from all the X-rays and scans, about these big spikes of bone right under my skin.

"What about the front of my pelvis?" I asked, fearful that both Brien and Klapper would refuse to investigate the painful bulge there, but determined to pursue my plan. "What about the long run for the short slide?"

"Oh, I'm your ally on that, now I've seen what happened inside," he replied.

"And Robert, what about the pin in my left arm?" I pressed.

"Well, is that a problem?" he asked. "Does it hurt?"

That was another moment of truth, when I knew the right answer.

"Yes," I said immediately.

"Then we'll take it out at the same time!"

The long run on my hidden path just added a few yards.

My file kept open, I was readmitted to TGIC, for non-physical therapies only, in time for my thirty-eighth birthday, which was celebrated with cake and candles, and new fellow clients. In therapy, Dr. Turner asked about my plans to return to work and teach at USC, and it fell to Jean to give me a tryout. I stood uncertainly at a whiteboard and described how the film and TV business worked to my fellow clients for all of fifteen minutes before my legs and concentration gave out. It did nothing for my self-confidence. How would I feel, my therapists asked, to volunteer as an English tutor to immigrants, and teach English as a second language?

The offer showed why it was risky to pursue unrealistic goals. The fastest possible return to work sounds good, but in my trip to Social Security, I dimly saw outlines of a trap. The system that saved my life seemed designed so I could use it for any purpose, other than to make a living.

For if I did, then the system would rule I wasn't disabled. And if I wasn't disabled, Great-West's insurance would end. I'd have to apply for regular health insurance, far beyond my means as an unpaid volunteer who taught English as a second language.

And that was beside the point in my case, because no health insurance company would offer me individual insurance anyway, not with a claims history that accelerated beyond the two million dollar mark, with no end in sight. I'd join the growing ranks of America's uninsured, unable to pay for the medical care I needed. "Pursue fitting for bilateral foot orthotics . . . ," my monthly TGIC report read. As their focus turned to a brace to make me walk faster, but no better, I fretted over my murky future. There was a nice ceremony at TGIC on my discharge in October. Jean hugged me goodbye.

"You keep that diary of your progress," she said, as she smiled and gave me TGIC's Final Discharge Report. She indicated one section of it that reviewed my cognitive and communication status, and described how I required three times the allowed time to complete a critical thinking test. So long after the crash, I still measured at the lowest percentile: my mental progress in that area barely begun.

As winter turned to spring, Dr. Brodney determined it was time for me to explore the recovery of those mental gaps. Where there was nothing before, his developmental optometry had helped recapture my lower peripheral vision on the left. This meant I no longer stumbled over unseen objects in my path, my vision loss now limited to the upper quadrant. I asked him why I still felt like I was alive in a dream, described the fractured landscape I saw around me that remained so unfamiliar.

"Brain injury affects vision in many different ways. You may have what's called 'blind sight,' Simon. You see things, but don't know you can."

That was a little beyond me, and said so. Ever patient, Alan gave it another shot.

"All of your vision still flows from your eyes into your brain, but perhaps part of your vision now routes into your subconscious—where your brain sees it, but can't consciously access it," he expanded. That seemed exactly right. I felt like I was stuck at that point between sleep and waking up, where your dream evolves incrementally, grows and extends with each iteration the way a dream does. And you cannot remember, or access it ever again, as you wake. Except that I was awake, and my brain was trapped there, consciously aware of this subconscious vision, unable to tap into it.

"I've taken you pretty much as far as I can until you're clear of surgery," Brodney added.

This was hard to hear when I still felt so much disconnect. Maybe he saw that in my face, because while I tried to think of something to say, he carried straight on.

"Normally this would be treated as your plateau," he continued, "but there's someone I know who I think can take you further." Dr. Lois Provda's specialty, he explained, was to rebuild minds.

When I arrived at the waiting room outside her office on L.A.'s Westside, she was with her last patient, so there was ample opportunity to read the gold- and silver-framed diplomas on her wall; the International Who's Who of Women certificate; the commendations from L.A. county school educators; and many other examples of her achievements.

I gradually became aware of a dark mop of hair that topped a young face. The face peered furtively at me around the frame of the office door, made no move, and remained there, visible only from the neck up. It was a ten-year-old boy, Lois's last patient, his session just ended.

"Hi!" I said, trying to break the silence.

The boy said nothing and continued to stare, unwilling to reveal any more of himself in the doorway. He adjusted his spectacles to get a better look at this patient nearly four times his age, and then scooted past me out the front door to a waiting parent in the street below.

I wasn't bothered by the age disparity between Lois's last patient and me—quite the opposite. Strokes and traumatic brain injuries know no boundaries, and as someone last measured at the bottom one percentile, I knew the moment I saw the boy's intent face that Brodney had sent me to the right place. I'd learn in due course he had a learning disability, and Lois was training his mind too.

An energetic woman with a warm and eager smile, she beckoned into her office as if inviting me into her home, except that the chairs set out ready for us across a work desk reminded me of the wooden ones for children. I was back to school in every sense.

Lois had an incredible variety of tests, which she pulled from a big cupboard set into the wall, like rabbits from a magician's hat. Her introductory puzzles seemed random except for one thing: I never felt so tired, so fast, in all my life. Her choices, and the order in which she administered them, she said, were designed to assess my attention, language, memory, problem-solving and visual-spatial abilities; my brain's visual and auditory sequencing. My mind resisted the load, the fatigue so great that Lois had to break her Neurobehavioral Status Exam into three sessions, to see whether or not I could benefit from cognitive retraining.

At the end of them, Lois reached her decision.

She would see me three times a week.

"You've made remarkable progress so far from the big injuries," she said. "Now, your mind and body need fine tuning."

I needed a lot of both. At my next visit to Dr. Klapper to assess progress, his X-rays showed the remaining hardware on the front of my pelvis and "no problems"— but they'd shown none on the back either. I felt like I knew nothing, had no mental capacity to figure whether it was right or wrong to continue.

"The therapists want me to wear an AFO on my leg so I can cross roads faster," I sighed. "I want to cross them *better*."

"Don't put a brace on your foot," Robert answered without hesitation. "Once you put it on, Simon, you'll never take it off."

His advice offered the challenge of every patient in search of the hidden path. Whether to stay the course, endure the risk of paralysis or death for the possibility of full recovery, or not. I weighed the choice of what to say about that possible next step.

"Your wound has healed properly this time," Dr. Klapper said with finality, as he ended our appointment. "Once you put it on, you'll never take it off" still echoed in my mind.

"Robert," I asked, my decision clear in that moment, "When would you be available to remove the front hardware?"

A month later, I checked in at Cedars before dawn for pre-op: on with the name tag; wheeled to a hospital room to strip into another hospital gown; and then up to Doctor Feelgood, dog-tired, heart hammering.

Dr. Klapper assembled a team of three surgeons this time, because to work his way so far inside me, he needed to coordinate the work of six skilled hands. Inescapably, I wondered if my quest for full recovery was to end with the medical dangers posed by, "Pelvis removal foreign body deep."

Laid bare once more on a gurney, it seemed crazy to second-guess my internist and Dr. Brien. Familiar sequence or not, I was terrified, and that was before I met Doctor *Feelbad*. I became aware that he'd fussed around for a while now, poked me several times with his needle to no apparent effect, other than to give me ample time to fill with doubt, clench first my jaw, and then my whole body, as I hit maximum stress.

It was ages since he asked the panic-trigger question, "And how much, Mr. Lewis, do you weigh?"

Thoughts of imminent death were displaced by more immediate questions, like what on earth he was up to, as he began to mutter to himself. "Hmm, that's . . . *interesting*. . . ." Beads of sweat formed in the suddenly clammy pre-op room.

"What's interesting?" I bleated. I'd lost all sensation in my arm.

"The vein actually has moved from where it should be," he mumbled.

A phrase came to me, one I used with crews on movie sets, where time is always critical.

"Tell me about the solution, not the problem," I gasped.

"Oh, I just got it in okay. It's . . . *interesting* is all."

I thought of my biker friend Zack's quite different word to describe it, until the IV's Demerol flowed, and took me down the slope of consciousness. When I came to in my hospital bed, a nurse folded my hand around a small control.

"This is a morphine button," she said. "Press it whenever the pain gets too much."

My internist came to examine me, and left happy. Dr. Klapper visited, and wasn't. The wound, he said, felt slightly warm to his touch, and warned I might not go home any time soon.

"It's a good thing we went in," he offered. "I've never seen anything like it—bone the size of a big lemon had grown right on top of your hardware!"

I marveled faintly how the body accommodated such a massive intruder.

"It can't," he answered. "The front of your pelvis is a vital part of the body, Simon."

I thought back to the exercise equipment of Cedars and TGIC, the effort to make me walk faster with a spiny, calcified lemon pressed against vital organs.

"You're very fortunate," he offered. "One wrong move and the bone growth could have ruptured you."

"Oh," I managed, as I resolved to listen to my body more, as best I could hear it.

Robert the whirlwind, I noticed, hadn't moved on. Clearly he wasn't done.

"There's something else. . . ." He paused. "That warmth . . . I think it's infection. If I'm right, the infection lived on your hardware, under the bone growth, feeding off your body."

"How could it live there undetected so long?" I asked, astonished.

"Because it was inside you, but *outside* your blood stream. That's why you've been so fatigued all the time. It was like a sealed cancer in you, and when we removed your hardware, we must have released it into your circulation. I'm sorry. . . ."

He slipped away. I hit my morphine button, and did the same.

The scheduled one-day stay extended to three weeks to battle the multi-resistant superbug, and as I lay once again at Cedars, kept alive by my IV, and last defense antibiotics, and morphine that coursed through my blood, my thoughts returned to that elusive track

I sought that might lead to full recovery. So far, at every step doctors uncovered and solved hidden problems; first the bone spikes, now a huge growth that harbored infection, all unseen until surgery.

It had worked to ignore the skull and bones posted at many of the turns, the "Death to all who pass here" warnings. As doctors added ever broader and more potent antibiotics to my IV, the more sense it made one day to remove my remaining hardware and not wait until it was "indicated by a symptom," like the doctors and nurses advised; follow the hidden path all the way while I was insured and young enough to take any risks that lay along it.

After discharge I was once again in Dr. Klapper's office, and by the time he arrived to discuss the surgery, I'd seen his operation report with its references to a slap hammer and mallet.

"Yes, it's pretty crude what we do in there all right," he laughed. "You know, there's nothing delicate about putting this stuff in, or taking it out. In medical school, I invented the device we use to remove old cement, which uses sound to break it up. Before that, we just chipped the old cement off with a hammer—even if some bone came away too!"

"How about the pin you took out of my arm?" I asked, still a bit shaken by his grizzly image.

"Patients always believe," Klapper said as he walked me over to the X-ray on a light panel, "that their surgeon does the operation, but often it's a resident, under supervision."

"But I always thought . . . ," I said, confused, "that my surgeon, who I see before I go to the hospital, is the one who operates on me."

"See what I mean?" he smiled. "Not in a teaching hospital. That's where doctors learn how to be surgeons—and the patient never knows!"

The logic was clear, but seemed impossible.

"How come none of us find out?" I puzzled.

"You agree to the substitution when you sign in."

I remembered the early morning admission forms that no scared, exhausted patient ever reads, or understands.

"Now that pin in your arm," he pointed to my X-ray, "was put in by a surgical resident in the intensive care unit who was being trained that night—not the surgeon." He tapped the white outline for emphasis. "I know because he put those anchor screws in the wrong place. He could have shattered the humerus the way he did it. And he left a hole in the muscle," Klapper added, with a smile, "that I sewed up, too, while I was in there!"

I was more grateful than ever that I found him, and that he did my surgery himself.

"Thank you," he said, "that's why I put together my own team. Only way I know for certain there'll be no substitutions is if I pick who's in the OR myself."

I knew this was my last chance.

"Do you think, Robert, you could one day make a team to take out my skull hardware?"

If doctors and therapists, with all their scans, missed bone spikes, a large lemon, and a hole in my arm, maybe they could overlook an elephant on my head. I said a silent prayer as I waited for his answer.

"Yes," he said after what seemed an eternity. "I know a neurosurgeon, Henry Stewart. He's a good man. If he recommends it, maybe I can team with him."

It was August by the time my insurance approved a consult, and I was in Dr. Stewart's clinic. Neurosurgeons are at the top of the medical hierarchy, which made it a long shot that this one might overrule Dr. Kern, whom he likely knew.

Dr. Stewart was young, remarkably so given that it takes ten years of graduate study to become a neurosurgeon to operate on brains and spines. His demeanor was very somber, very distant as he studied his freshly ordered CT of my skull.

"Removal of this hardware may be medically reasonable, but it's not medically necessary," he began. My heart sank.

"Also, since your skull is only eighty percent fused, there are serious risks to any surgery on it," he continued. Now my heart plummeted, as Stewart reasoned hope away.

"For example," he explained gravely, "if I remove the plates when these scans show fusion is incomplete, there's a risk your cranioplasty will become unstable."

He cleared his throat, and then adopted the tone doctors use to tell a patient their consultation is over, his "final opinion" voice.

"I recommend you wait at least another eighteen to twenty-four months for it to fuse completely," he said, "and we'll review it then."

As 1998 began and I waited for my skull to fuse on Dr. Stewart's timetable, my brother David recommended a foot specialist, who referred me to a Dr. Rose, who wasn't sure why I came in, but was friendly as he reviewed the images and files my mother assembled for the consultation.

The medical language of his report was hard to follow, but his conclusion was not. "At this point," Dr. Rose wrote, "Mr. Lewis appears to be a good candidate for a SPLATT procedure." A SPLATT, he explained, would surgically split my ankle tendons, and he had another procedure in mind for me too. He noticed how my toes clenched involuntarily. Babies do this until their brains learn how to release them. In brain injury, the path can be damaged. Rather than see if my brain could relearn it, Dr. Rose had a different prescription.

"I can fix that. Snip, snip, no problem!" he said several times in the consultation.

"Won't that weaken my foot?" I asked.

"Oh no, you don't need them for balance," he said, with the good cheer of a surgeon who likes nothing more, when all is said and done, than to operate.

"All it means is you'll never pick up pencils with your toes again!"

He wanted to split and transfer my ankle tendons and snip others in my toes, while a second opinion surgeon wanted to extend another. By making a small nick in my Achilles tendon, he explained, "just like into the edge of a rubber band," it would allow the tendon to stretch, the muscle to which it attached to relax, and help me walk.

To solve my confusion, my ever-helpful neighbor Harry recommended I get a third opinion from a top internist. You could feel efficiency and certainty in the air when I arrived at the plush Beverly Hills medical office building, and was ushered into a very chic waiting room. I was impressed by the leather bound Harvard Medical School yearbook strategically placed in the center of his bookshelf, and recognized the youthful doctor from his TV appearances as a medical expert when he strode in. He said he'd reviewed my files and wanted to hear my questions.

I explained them as quickly as I could, from what I could do about the elephant that lived on my head to the critical questions about my pelvis; why I couldn't walk and the recommendation of three different tendon surgeries. I finished with how I would follow any course of treatment he recommended. Now for some answers from the Harvard man, I thought. The expert would tell me what to do, which medical tests would decide which surgery was best.

"Be grateful for what you have. You're lucky to be alive," was his diagnosis.

I fared better with a sports specialist Harry also suggested.

"That's a bit of a mystery," Dr. Whittaker said.

I was at his clinic in Santa Monica. He'd welcomed me in, taken an X-ray of my pelvis on his own equipment without delay, and immediately examined it for himself. If my experience was typical, in which radiologists missed so much, then maybe the best doctors relied on their own equipment and their own eyes, and Dr. Whittaker was chief orthopedist for one of the biggest professional sports teams in L.A.

"Um, yes, I see," I replied.

It was an aspiration more than a corroboration. What I really meant was that I *wished* I could see the "bit of a mystery" amongst the hazy lines of my pelvis, that was now beautifully free of titanium plates. But Dr. Whittaker could tell me no more about the mystery or how to solve it.

In July, I was an usher at my brother Jonathan's marriage to Elinor, a vivacious and successful executive with Chase Bank. Whether this made me feel better, or simply boosted my morale, I finally was ready to follow the long-overdue recommendation of a kind nurse to her cousin as my new dentist. He was a solo practitioner in the San Fernando Valley, conveniently near our home, who turned out to be young, friendly, and cheerful. After X-rays, he disappeared and a beautiful hygienist started to clean my teeth, an angel in more ways than one. As she heard my story and worked, she told me about the course of treatment planned for me. "Whaa . . . whaad . . . *fillingssh?*" I gabbled through Mr. Slurpy, and a mouthful of dental gear.

"Here, see those red dots?" she asked sweetly, and held up the X-rays to make sure I could.

"Those are all the places Doctor says your teeth need fillings."

I saw red dots in more ways than one. There must have been fifteen or twenty of them. Maybe recommendations to family members who want to build their dental practice could work, but this felt like a "drill, fill, and bill" situation.

"And I can also improve the color of your teeth!" young Doctor Red Dots promised, as I stumbled out into the sunlight, my teeth clean, and still intact.

I waited as best I could like Stewart instructed, and saw Dr. Klapper in December, in hopes of a different solution to my constant pain. It occurred to me that even with the titanium pin removed and the hole in my muscle repaired, my left shoulder still hurt. Maybe the pain and pressure there were linked somehow with the elephant on my head. It was impossible to believe anything remained the doctors had missed, but I pressed him for a shoulder MRI. He looked at it a long time.

"That dark area," he said finally. "I think that's blood."

So the new year found me back at Cedars. Perched on a chair at half past six in the morning, handed the inevitable plastic bag for clothes.

For this procedure, Dr. Klapper special ordered a cold-water jacket to help my shoulder heal. It would be in my hospital room, ready for nurses to apply and reduce inflammation as soon as I woke. I was well taken care of, I reflected, as I gazed at the plastic clothes bag and remembered how I was told to undress, except no one came for ages. How then I sat in my flimsy gown, starved from having fasted since the night before, until a transportation nurse finally showed up with warm blankets, to wheel me into pre-op.

I couldn't help but ask myself what would happen if I *wasn't* ready when transportation came. To see,

I half-changed and put my sweats jacket on over the flimsy. It's amazing how dehumanized you feel without your clothes; how much better, warm, and comfortable I felt with some still on. The nurse seemed surprised when he showed more than half an hour later.

"No hurry," he said, as I slipped off pants and top and went straight under the blankets, warm, relaxed, and ready for Feelgood.

I learned another lesson when I first regained consciousness. Just as I was to be wheeled from the OR to the recovery room, a group trauma came in. Instantaneously, my level of care dropped to zero. A nurse hurriedly pushed my wheelchair into a corner of the nearest empty room, locked the wheels, and disappeared.

I was completely trussed, plugged in with IV and catheter, and the nurse hadn't had time to reunite me with my glasses. Maybe Feelgood's drugs had something to do with it too, but after half an hour fixated on a blank wall inches in front of me, during which it became clear I was abandoned and forgotten, I broke down. I started to count numbers, the last level of neglected misery I learned at Cedars.

As even more time passed, I began to call "help" after each count, and got a little more desperate, a little louder, each time. It wasn't out of weakness or politeness; there were limits to how much sound I could make with a catheter inserted down below, and didn't want to find out what they were.

Finally, a nurse happened to pass by the doorway at the right moment.

"Can I help you?"

"I . . . have brain injury—and I'm having a breakdown," I sobbed.

In seconds, I was wheeled the few yards that separated me from my waiting family, who'd asked repeatedly where I was, as soon as I inexplicably disappeared from the operating room, yet not shown up in recovery.

"Right again! It was a good thing we went into your shoulder," Robert smiled happily.

I was safely back in his clinic with Bibi, Mark, the portrait of Wilt, and the great fish, serenely undisturbed in their tank. Dr. Klapper was exuberant.

"I filled *two* surgical buckets with the blood and debris that came out of your shoulder! The MRI documented impingement, and now that I've released it, we can see your rotator cuff is intact!"

I wondered how I could have done so many exercises recommended by prior therapists, and believed they helped my shoulder, when instead they built up massive internal damage—the tubs Klapper filled with debris. As I looked back, I suddenly realized how there was some kind of mental black hole at work within me that sucked away awareness of my problems. My brain didn't know what fell into the black hole, what it either couldn't see or feel. I literally didn't know what I was missing. And as Dr. Klapper's latest success drained debris from my system, I felt the surge; started to feel less tired as another 24/7 supply of toxins to my blood stream abated.

He next recommended outpatient therapy at his hospital.

"But Robert, that didn't help when I was discharged from Cedars the first time," I pointed out.

"It's all new," he said. "We've a special physiatry program called Where East Meets West. Go see Michelle Banning."

Dr. Michelle Banning, a young, sincere rehab specialist, encouraged me when I visited her clinic. One of her partners was on my original Cedars team. He remembered my case, she explained, and authored one of the chapters in the medical school textbook used across the U.S.—the chapter devoted to head injury.

"According to the textbook, Simon," she said with a smile, "your recovery so far, given the extent of your brain damage, is *miraculous.*"

It was great to hear her say it, better still to know that nearly five years after the crash, Dr. Banning thought I could improve further with extensive rehab, as she started me on a very Eastern-influenced course of detoxification: Traumeel injections, tendon sheath and ligament massages, Lymphomyosot drops in water, Gelsemium Homaccord, and doses of Galium-Heel. As she worked on me, Dr. Banning shared her approach to long-term care, and how patients healed differently. Some with stroke enjoyed full recovery, others permanently lost use of their limbs, and no one knew exactly why, any more than I knew each day how I would feel.

"Miraculous progress so far is wonderful, Dr. Banning," I said in a moment of clarity during a treatment, "but what more can I do?"

"I could send you to Master Kim," she answered. "I've had brain-injured patients make real advances using Tai Chi, and Tae Kwon Do."

It appeared there were three tests I must undergo before she'd medically approve me even to attempt Master Kim's therapy. I saw the neurologist first, who gave some standard vision tests, but never discussed any way to image my nerves or how to help them.

For the second Western test, I saw a specialist in Beverly Hills for another EMG of my lower body, but he too found nothing treatable, and his report made no reference to the mystery Dr. Whittaker saw in my pelvis. Both doctors confirmed the sad limitations of neurology diagnosis, how little they could tell me about either my peripheral nerves or my brain.

And then came the third and final test before I could meet Master Kim. I was in Dr. Henry Stewart's office once again, to see him for the first time since he told me it wasn't either safe or necessary to remove my skull hardware. He reviewed my file carefully.

"Yeah," he sighed hesitantly, "it's probably worth checking your spine to see if the problem in your leg comes from there."

"I've no problem with a spinal myelogram," I assured, when asked. It sounded similar to an EMG, and didn't see how it could be any more unpleasant.

"Any precautions?" I asked Stewart's receptionist, as I scheduled my appointment at Cedars-Sinai Imaging. Perhaps you weren't supposed to eat before the test.

"You may want to lie down and rest after," was her sunny reply.

As a radiologist performed my "injection for lumbar myelogram; CT reconstruction," I felt weird numbness spread through the center of my body—which was okay as it meant no conscious pain—when he told me to lean in different directions, and I tried to ignore the spinal tap in me. Nonetheless, it felt as though my spine somehow lost its flexibility. The sensation reminded me of a surgical IV, but mixed in were misgivings I never felt before. Far down the slope of consciousness, a monster stirred.

I went to bed as soon as we got home that afternoon, as the nurse and instruction sheet from Cedars Imaging recommended. To be on the safe side, my parents placed a bell on my bedside table. I never fell asleep but simply lay there, aware of how I felt progressively worse, as something from the core of my being roiled, and gathered force.

We watched Kenneth Branagh's *Hamlet* the night before, to take my mind off the test, and, as the attack began around 3:00 AM, I felt calm when I rang my emergency bell. Except my parents, fast asleep, didn't hear. Then the full assault began.

My head was about to explode, and I desperately needed to pull my eyes out of their sockets, anything to release the pressure inside my skull. My central nervous system erupted into full revolt, my arms and legs almost shut down. I had to act before it was too late. Two desperate, shaky half-steps got me closer toward the bedroom door, where I rang frantically until I heard my parents wake, then collapsed onto the bed just as my legs went rigid and I lost control.

The seizure progressed in the seconds it took my mother and father to reach me. By then my arms too were rigid as I frantically gestured "up" at my legs, which they raised onto a suitcase my father grabbed. He dialed the emergency number on the instructions sheet, except Cedars Imaging gave us an old one, with a number that was out of service. It made no difference. Whatever happened next would do so long before any ambulance could reach us.

As I gasped for air and hyperventilated, my brain released every drop of adrenaline; its last attempt to wrest back control of my lungs as the attack reached my diaphragm. No matter how hard I wrenched my body, I knew I couldn't get air into my lungs if the diaphragm went as rigid as my arms and legs, and I would suffocate. Already the only sound I could make was a tortured, shallow death wheeze; a literal last gasp, which is how most of us die.

It was harder for my parents than for me. I'd lived in the shadow of death, and felt acceptance; had just watched Hamlet in the movie, contemplate the end of his life.

To be or not to be, that is the question.

Either the attack would reach my heart and lungs and stop them, or they'd bear me through. My heart pounded furiously past all limits, it felt like a hundred and sixty or more.

If it be now, 'tis not to come;
If it be not to come, it will be now;
If it be not now, yet it will come:
*   the readiness is all. . . .*

Our mortality, our final moment of life, will come. It was true, and I was ready. I could sense the mountains I saw in my coma, the monsters stir again within, the villagers who waited to welcome my return. But the attack finally abated. What remained was the worst headache I ever experienced. From this unbearable pain, doctors produced a 3-D holograph reconstruction of my lower spine, and a report that, I anticipated, would be the greatest wisdom available in modern medicine. "Partial fusion left sacroiliac joint? Is this . . . ?" were its final words, the unanswered questions a token of all that remained unknown.

"What was *that*?" I asked Dr. Stewart when I finally made it to his clinic, glad of the opportunity to see him again and keep my case alive.

"We call them spinal headaches—but we really don't know what they are," he offered candidly. "Get them in maybe five percent of cases. But your reaction was . . . unusual."

Even if the tests couldn't diagnose me, I was grateful for their confirmation that I could attempt a course of Tae Kwon Do, the Korean martial art.

Beverly Hills Martial Arts was a well-appointed facility with a padded floor, wall mirrors, and handrails all around. Bong C. Kim—Grand Master Kim—was a very friendly, and extremely intense man in his early thirties. Dr. Banning, he confirmed, had sent other patients. With that briefest explanation, his eyes fixed me with a courteous, unwavering focus in his dojo.

"We start. Now."

He gestured to the floor, after a formal bow that

I copied. It didn't seem possible my left leg could support my weight, and I asked whether my ankles would capsize when I put on the floppy soft shoes worn by his students and tried to stand on the padded floor.

"We start . . . *now*," answered my grand master.

So began my first experience of Tae Kwon Do in a private session, as Master Kim patiently guided my body into a balanced stance, explained how important it was I find my center, find the right way to breathe. I went every weekday, the sessions intense, from a warm-up focused on smooth gentle motions, to calisthenics, to *hyung*—drills made up of prearranged patterns of foot-kicks and hand-punches—which integrated both the physical and philosophical elements of Tae Kwon Do. The goal, Master Kim said, as I struggled with the most rigorous routine so far demanded of me, was to achieve total mind and body control, not necessarily physically, but instead by full awareness of the world around me with uncompromising spiritual honesty.

The issue of compromise presented itself at home one evening when I saw that *Look Who's Talking*, my biggest hit and first film for a major studio, was on TV, but without my credit. In Hollywood, those credits in the main titles are a big deal, inclusion of my name in them of vital importance to me. But, as if I no longer existed, my name was gone from the film's opening, where the voice of Bruce Willis cheerleads the sperm on their merry way to conception. I faced the critical question of whether I was still a complete and effective person able to take steps to remedy this, or a disabled person who couldn't, who must accept that I was out of the business.

The philosophy of Tae Kwon Do, its lifetime-long perspective, brought me the answer. No matter how long my recovery took, the day might come when I'd define myself as a man who could write and produce movies, influence his environment, and find full recovery, even if I didn't know when. I called a lawyer, an old friend, and the ultimate resolution included worldwide recall and correction of my producer credit on the film and DVD, a Hollywood first.

Several weeks into my Tae Kwon Do program, as I lay face down on the padded floor of his dojo, Master Kim stepped one foot onto my pelvis, tried carefully to free it deeper within, then back with his hands, and then the foot once more; I could tell he was unhappy.

"What is it?" I said indistinctly, grateful the padded floor cushioned my face.

"Something *wrong*. . . . No right with bone. . . . Ask Banning."

Master Kim was totally focused on something he could feel, maybe something the Western machines couldn't see and missed along with the cliffhanger questions that ended my last spine report.

"Master Kim wants to know *exactly*: What's this area, where he feels something wrong?" I asked Dr. Banning at our next appointment, careful to use his exact words at the martial arts dojo. I pointed to where Master Kim's foot had probed deep.

"Is it calcification?"

Dr. Banning monitored my progress with Master Kim closely, but she had no firm answers that day, beyond recommendation of some additional exercises that, she said, were used by ballet dancers to fine train their feet.

"Do you think it's related to what Dr. Whittaker called a *bit of a mystery* in my pelvis?" I pressed for what could possibly remain in there after all the hardware was taken out.

"I think it comes down to the most potent medicine of all, Simon," she evaded. "Tincture of time."

That Presidents' Day weekend, my family had

brunch at Shutters on the Beach, a Santa Monica hotel with a sweeping view of the Pacific Ocean. We sat and pondered what to do next, if Dr. Banning was done with me.

"Well, look who's here!" called out two voices, friendly and unmistakable.

It was Joy and Harvey Warren, also by the ocean for brunch. We seemed bound by fate for them to come to my rescue. For as we updated them on all the surgeries and tests since they visited me at Cedars, and the limited answers we found so far, Joy told me something she never mentioned when I was her manager.

"My brother's a nuclear radiologist," she said.

Dr. Shelton was a retired Air Force Colonel who became interested in the field during his medical training in the military, specialized in it after discharge, and was now Chief of Nuclear Medicine at the medical school of the University of California, at Davis.

Dr. Shelton opened his schedule and two days later, my mother and I landed in Sacramento for the short taxi ride to his clinic. It was my first experience with the SPECT scan, or single photon emission computed tomography, as a nurse explained she'd inject a radioactive isotope. I was still surprisingly afraid of needles, and said so.

"Don't worry," she smiled, "We use a baby butterfly—it's the smallest we have."

I hardly felt it, and then braced myself. Whether the sensors were crackling needles like an EMG, the spinal tap of a myelogram, or electrodes glued to my shaved scalp like the EEG, nerve tests were always very nasty, and hurt a whole lot.

"Will you strap me down so I won't shake?" I asked.

"Goodness, no!" she laughed. "You just lie there and don't move."

It's remarkable how much you want to twitch every muscle in your body when someone says that. But I lay motionless as instructed, and reflected how I always assumed that the more painful a test, the deeper the information it must yield. To lie still under this silent black device after a painless injection didn't seem likely to provide much in the way of clues; it was way too easy.

Especially when, twenty minutes later, Dr. Shelton was ready to show his images. The typed report, he explained, would follow by mail.

"Here's your brain injury . . . and here . . . and here," he pointed. "The damage is much more extensive than the Cedars MRI showed."

Worse than I feared, but Shelton started his diagnosis with the bad news.

"But," he continued, "your motor strip—which controls your muscles—has only minimal encroachment. If the infarct extended just one half centimeter more, you'd be paralyzed down the left side of your body."

Half my body had survived by five millimeters. I thought of my hearing, and the bone the size of a grasshopper's leg that preserved it. There was so much I was grateful for, and Dr. Shelton's images confirmed the diagnosis of my original neurologist at Cedars. Full motor function should return. Shelton's opinion came down on that side of the critical question, with objective data.

I knew my mother's next question before she spoke.

"Then, why can't he walk?"

"My first doctor at Cedars thought it was something curable," I tried.

"Yes, possibly in the spine or pelvis," Shelton answered. "Look for evidence of bony entrapment on the pelvic floor."

Shelton's written report was phrased with all

the caution I expected, to the effect that it was *"plausible* that your pelvic fractures *may* have resulted in scarring along the pelvic floor, *potentially* resulting in your symptoms." But his painless test yielded some of the best information, and potentially revealed the next steps along the hidden path. As Lois Provda continued to fine tune my mind with therapies designed to integrate the different components within it, I felt I'd found the best doctors that spring. Even as I coped with bouts of Dracula eye and the elephant on my head, I was, I thought, on the path to full recovery aided by the best doctors and treatments in Western medicine.

As soon as we returned to L.A., my mother and I visited Dr. Klapper for a follow-up. He was an excellent diagnostician, I reflected.

"No sign of any more infection. Your shoulder and pelvis have healed beautifully," he said.

He turned back to us from the light panel.

"Simon, the sky's the limit!"

"But why can't he walk?" my mother pleaded again.

Robert said he'd seen eighteen patients that day, as he ran his hand through his hair. I noticed he looked tired, but he always came through for me, and the answer to my mother's question, the question raised by the SPECT scan, was the key to the next step on the path.

"My theory on *that*," Robert said after a long pause, "is that there's pressure on your spinal cord. Somewhere after it leaves the base of your spine, before it enters your leg and becomes your sciatic nerve."

He answered my next question before I asked.

"If you were a woman, maybe, but a man's pelvis is too narrow, Simon. There's no safe way. And even if I went in, I wouldn't know what I was looking for."

I thought about those few inches between the

bottom of my spine and top of my leg, where perhaps the answer waited hidden, and had to ask.

"Do you know anyone who could, Robert?"

There was a long silence, and when he spoke, it was with unmistakable finality.

"Maybe you could get a cowboy surgeon to try. But remember the good news. Right now, Simon, when you look down, you see a left leg. I can't tell you about your phone lines—your nerves—but your pelvis is all set."

And there was silence in the consultation cubicle.

Dr. Klapper was done with my pelvis and me, far short of full recovery. I was shocked, but doctors aren't like Sherlock Holmes, sleuths who find every clue and perfectly solve the mystery. I knew that from all the missed information on X-rays and MRIs. I'd learned something else, too; also unlike Sherlock Holmes, doctors and therapists weren't proactive.

Their role was to fix people, not save them. Not suggest things that *might* be wrong, or anticipate surgeries I might need because of complications that *could happen*. It was to wait for a problem to reach a level where I complained about it, and sought their help.

There was something else I noticed about their different fields of expertise. If they weren't too proactive within their specialty, they also stayed very close to it, and offered little advice or suggestions outside of it. I began to think of doctors as if I was on an uncertain trip through a supermarket that was filled with their wares. The storefront sign read "Shop 'Til You Drop . . . Or Recover." But unlike a regular store, where you easily find everything you need, in this supermarket everything was either random, or it was organized but labeled in a language I didn't understand.

And unlike Wal-Mart greeters who gladly point you to where to find everything you need, no doctor was likely to tell me what was available on any other aisle in the store but their own.

Nothing helped fill the silence after he warned us that any further pelvic surgery would be by a cowboy, and I could lose my left leg.

"Robert," my mother implored, "isn't there anyone who can see where the nerve is pressed?"

More silence followed.

"There's someone at Rancho Los Amigos," he eventually said, "people call 'the guru of gait.' Come back with the report."

CHAPTER THIRTEEN

FALSE PROPHETS

Things at the worst will cease
Or else climb upward. . . .
　　　　—William Shakespeare,
　　　　Macbeth, act 4, scene 2

In Greek mythology, destiny depended on the Three Fates, three ladies seated at a spinning wheel, where they spun the thread of our existence and determined our futures. They were a merry trio. Our feeble attempts to cheat them and extend our time on Earth made them laugh because they always prevailed.

　　Did the ancients know things we've forgotten? I wondered, as I gazed out from the car. Fields of brown and green passed by in the early morning sun, as we drove south to Rancho Los Amigos. My condition was stable, but so was the constant elephant on my head. I'd relative youth and determination in my favor, but wondered how much thread the Fates had spun for me in that precious woven skein of theirs. For the thread our Greek ancestors believed in turned out to be our double helix of DNA, and right then I felt as if my doctors were no more in control of my recovery than if it was still in the hands of those happy women at their wheel.

Rancho Los Amigos Medical Center was a facility with a mission, Robert told me, to help polio patients to walk. We drove in past what looked like Second World War-era bungalows, and were issued a plastic blue card at the front gate.

It wasn't quite so organized in the cavernous lobby, where I saw a man on crutches at the reception counter.

"You operated on me six weeks ago!" he shouted at the top of his voice. "What do you mean you can't find my file?!"

His desperate wail started to break, and fell into the distance as we were led down a hallway to the clinic, where a nurse handed me a form with an outline of the human body. "Mark where you have pain or numbness," it requested. I covered the picture with arrows and circles, and then waited in hope of answers from the Guru. I didn't meet her, but instead was prepped and ushered into a long narrow studio.

It was bathed in ultra violet light and I saw video cameras set into the ceiling around the room, ready to record my motion and stride. In my prep, a nurse took long needles, with sensors about the size of ping-pong balls at one end, and stuck them into my nerves at the other. It was almost as though it was the pain that made them glow bright blue in the eerie light. On my feet she strapped loose sandals with more needle sensors. I stood in my flimsy, vaguely aware of the walls of computers, and waited while lab techs announced my case information, their voices unearthly as they were amplified through the studio speakers.

"Extensors, left," one intoned. I dreaded what might happen next.

"Walk," another said.

I hobbled forward, pins with balls weirdly aglow, wires suspended from the end of them. The pain was awful, so I tried to focus on each step. My brain wouldn't. Instead, an extraneous thought surged up the slope of consciousness from nowhere, Johnny Cash's song, "I Walk The Line," but the words escaped me as I looked at my unsteady feet that could do no such thing.

"Go faster," the tech called, detached, his voice reverberating in the studio as he worked through his tests. I hobbled even worse as pain surged, computer drives hummed and whirred, and more unrelated thoughts birthed inside me as I began to lose control. After the needles were mercifully out, Dr. Polk joined my parents in his office to discuss the initial findings of his dynamic EMG of my left lower extremity.

"Good news!" he began. "There's no need to go on wearing a brace on your leg to walk."

"But I've not worn one," I replied. "Robert said if I put one on, I'd never take it off."

That didn't sway him. He turned to my parents.

"This long after the crash, we know for sure that Simon's leg weakness is from his brain injury. It's permanent and won't improve, but he can live without a brace."

"What would be involved?" my father wanted to know.

"We call it a SPLATT, a tendon transfer to balance his foot," Dr. Polk repeated the prescription of the specialist who was ready to "snip, snip" my toes, except there was more to come.

"I must do *two* SPLATTs," Dr. Polk expanded, "and he'll still limp because there's no appropriate tendon to use on his third problem."

I wondered about all those circles and arrows I marked on the outline of my body, and the multiple surgeries that would require, Polk explained, "several months of rehab."

"Can you help my pelvis and upper leg? The *whole* of my left leg?" I asked.

"I don't know about that, but I can fix your left ankle," he replied.

I thought about the desperate man I heard in the lobby, the disconnect between "months of rehab" by a facility, and the fact it could forget a patient after only six weeks, especially as, once done, tendon transfers are irreversible. On that, Dr. Polk was also clear.

"*Long-term*, how many tendons do I have?" I tried. "I mean in a few years' time, if my body changes, would you need to adjust them again? Retune my body like a guitar?"

"I really don't think so," came the reply. "But the benefits should last. When do you want to come in?"

"We're in no hurry," said my father. "In the next few months perhaps."

"If you do nothing," Polk added, "Simon will end up confined to a wheelchair. How about in six weeks?"

When the detailed report arrived at our home, there were pages of computer printout, and a letter, apparently from the guru, that described a "challenging pattern of abnormal muscle control," made a definite diagnosis that after five years my brain would heal no more, and concluded with the recommendation of several tendon transfers as the best and only way to fix my body.

When I asked my internist, he could not dispute the findings and prognosis. My instinct was to postpone, but I was equally reluctant to put off procedures that promised to save me from a wheelchair.

"They want to book the surgery in six weeks.

What do you think?" I asked Lois at my next session.

"Tell me the date, Simon . . . ," she spoke deliberately, "so I'll know when to lie down in the drive in front of your home, and stop you leaving for the hospital."

I still didn't know the right choice when I returned to Robert Klapper with Rancho's report.

"They want to schedule my surgery in six weeks," I began at my appointment, as Robert scanned the pages, "but I never met the guru. . . ."

He took me through to his private office, with patents on the wall awarded for his inventions that advanced orthopedic medicine.

"Simon, there's so much we don't know," he began. "Take electrical stimulation of the nerves, that was used in Eastern medicine for hundreds of years, but long ignored here in the West."

I remembered sessions of it at Cedars; how current ran through my left arm, and the sensation helped my brain learn how to move it.

"That's right," Klapper agreed. "And guess what? Now, it's used by everyone. And no one knows how it works!"

He talked about an American-trained Chinese doctor who got remarkable results for her patients. It sounded like a good lead, but I reminded Robert I was nearly at Dr. Stewart's recommended threshold of eighteen months. The SPECT scan in Sacramento—the images that showed everywhere that the elephant in my head could hide—increased my desperate resolve to remove the plates in my skull.

"I could probably work with Henry Stewart if he recommends something," Robert pondered, as we parted.

"Your clinical presentation and my recommendation haven't changed," Dr. Stewart flatly stated his opinion, as he viewed fresh scans in his clinic. "Your skull remains unstable, and it's dangerous to attempt surgery before fusion is complete."

I stood before him, desperate to move my recovery to the next level, but didn't see how when he just said *no*.

"But it's getting on for two years, and I still feel like there's an elephant on my head," I repeated brokenly, like a child. I was close to tears as my last chance faded, before a final plea.

"Robert said he'd make a team . . . ," I tried.

It wasn't what Klapper said—more like what I wished he had—anything for the chance to be free of my elephant. Dr. Stewart seemed somewhat surprised, too, that Dr. Klapper would make such an offer. I was on thin ice, with too much at stake to care.

"Really? I'll speak to him," was all Stewart said.

In spite of its risks, a faint possibility for this option remained, pursued with an emergency call to Klapper on our cell phone as soon as my mother and I were outside. Bibi put me straight through.

"Robert! Henry will only do it if *you* form the team. He's calling you right now."

"Oh . . . okay," he answered.

In June, I was back at Cedars, head shaved once more to the scalp, for Dr. Stewart, with Dr. Klapper at his side, to remove my skull hardware.

Unlike the plates and screws in my jaw, arm, and pelvis, the eight Leibinger miniplates and their screws in my skull were small and delicate, with bone formed all around them.

With Dr. Klapper beside him, Henry Stewart began to cut through the layers of my scalp to expose my skull and the titanium plates. It went well as his steady hands removed the screws that secured the first plate, lifted it free, and paused to check if my skull held fast. The second plate went the same.

The first tiny screw on the third plate was encased in bone, and resisted. When he tried again to turn it, the titanium shaft sheared off.

Dr. Stewart dropped the broken screw head into the specimen container and did the only thing he could; he moved on to the next.

"Wait!" Klapper said above my unconscious head. "We need to get the shaft of that screw out. To get the plate—"

"We leave it," Stewart said tersely.

My skull was completely exposed. As lead surgeon, with one eye always on the operating room clock, he needed to move on to the fourth plate and get to the halfway mark.

"No, Henry," Klapper insisted calmly, "it's not just medical, it's *spiritual*. This guy's gonna wake up and ask, 'Did you get it all?' And I'm gonna tell him, 'Yes, it's *all* out of your head!'"

There was the shortest of silences.

"You've got exactly five minutes, Robert," Stewart relented. "Go."

Klapper was right, of course. That was exactly what I asked him post-operatively, which is how I learnt what went down in the OR.

"So I started to excavate bone from your skull as quick as I could, to get that screw shaft," Klapper would tell me. "With your brain right there in front of me!"

When the skull hardware was finally out, the team copiously irrigated the entire area with antibiotics, and closed me up.

I opened my eyes, this time in a hospital room that looked like a small apartment. A social worker at Cedars recognized my mother and, as I was something of a hospital regular, found an empty suite for us, which was kind.

In a handheld mirror, I saw my eyes were Drac-

ula-red again, and wondered if this hardware was infected too, the infection flushed into my eyes during its
removal.

I would ask Alan Brodney the next time I saw him
for vision therapy, and he'd say there was no way infection could flow from the hardware to my eyes, as they're
sealed units. And then I'd begin to think my body had
unknown pathways; that maybe invincible bugs lived
on them, remembering how returning astronauts found
microbes that survived on the U.S. flag on the moon,
even in the vacuum of space. Maybe some lived on in
the same way, invulnerably sealed inside my skull.

But that morning after skull surgery, I simply
told Dr. Stewart when he visited how much I hoped this
was my final Dracula eye, and this problem was rooted
out of my head once and for all.

"How do you feel?" he asked.

"Not too bad," I lied. Truth to tell, I wasn't sure
how I felt. The brain surgery left a tear in the fabric of
my consciousness.

"You can go home, if you like," he added improb-
ably.

The car ride home was searingly painful and I'd
not step outside my parents' house for five weeks, but
when I made it to Dr. Stewart's clinic, he couldn't wait
to show me the old CT scans.

"It was fascinating," Stewart began, excited. "You
see how your skull was fractured here . . . and here . . .
and here . . . and here?"

I wished I could find it in me to match his enthusiasm about the gray and white jagged lines across
whole sections of my skull.

"Kern did a great job with those eight plates," he
pressed on.

Truthfully, I wasn't sure what he could see, and
the sight of my crushed skull still unnerved me too

much to speak.

"You see, Simon," Stewart filled the silence, "the fractures created an island in your skull. The plates Kern installed were like little bridges across . . . ," he carefully began to draw pencil marks to demonstrate, "that connected to the island from every side—to hold that section of your skull in place while it fused."

I thought I saw what he meant. There was the area of my skull ringed around completely by fractures; a separate island in my head surrounded by little titanium bridges.

"They worked to the point," Stewart went on, "that you were eighty percent fused, but the hardware continued to hold the island in a fixed position. At that point, they stopped your recovery and prevented final fusion. Perhaps that was why you felt an elephant was on your head. It was incredible. When I opened you, I saw stress lines in your skull from the pressure!"

If head injuries and skull fractures were so common, I wondered why no doctor mentioned this possibility before its discovery in the operating room.

"The CT scan couldn't show me that," Stewart explained, "because stress lines don't show up." That sounded like pretty essential information for all the people with broken heads.

"Maybe someone should do a research project into it," Stewart agreed thoughtfully. "Where there's an island fracture, the hardware may need to come out."

I wondered if the research would ever be done; about all the patients in the world forced to live with elephants on their heads, but it was time to thank Dr. Stewart for his skill and move on.

I wish I could say my release brought total relief, but with the elephant gone, my head was filled with silence. My brain felt like it was dead again, returned to the first singularity that is within us—our point of origin—from which everything our minds will become is built. By day, I rested in bed with no sound, blinds shut tight, and felt overwhelmed, as if the elephant's release undammed a torrent of sensations that flooded every nerve in my body, a million billion intercellular conversations that I could not hear, and no machine could detect. Long nights passed the same way.

It was the early fall of 1999. Medical insurance policies typically run for the calendar year, and as summer advances, insurance companies and employers make decisions about what health coverage they will offer their policy holders, usually to start from an effective date of the following January 1. I could barely focus my eyes when, with relief, I signed Prudential Health Care's Enrollment Form when it came in the mail, and my first check cleared, coverage locked for the following year.

President Clinton had signed HIPAA into law, legislation that addressed the plight of people forced to turn down jobs because they couldn't get into a new employer's group plan. Under HIPAA rules, if a person left one group health plan, and applied for another, the new group had to accept the application and provide coverage.

Right then, I didn't know about or need the new rules. With insurance confirmed, Dr. Shelton's SPECT scan appeared the only road map back to the hidden path, and Dr. Klapper the one clinician still ready to investigate and operate, but only if an image captured and diagnosed the elusive "evidence of bony entrapment on the pelvic floor."

"I'll call the radiologist and make sure he sees you himself," he agreed.

On the day, a tech fitted my headset, slid me into the machine's little tunnel, and I settled back to the sounds of the MRI; the cloppety-clop of the first horse's hooves as they clattered by my head, a second lone horse, a pause, and then the stampede.

As the session advanced, I wondered what became of the promised radiologist who, with the detailed guidance of Dr. Shelton's SPECT scan, would find a critical clue. Except the radiologist didn't appear, and his final report, after the list of organs he scanned and found problem free, also confirmed that my gallbladder was "*unremarkable.*" I might have felt more confident about his conclusion had he noticed my once gangrenous gallbladder was no longer there.

The MRI triggered an emergency conference call from the insurance company. Having received the forms and accepted my check, Prudential Insurance denied payment for that MRI, and more broadly would not insure me. Every year the business of caring ends recovery treatments this way for millions of sick and disabled. My situation looked hopeless. After the false assurance of coverage, I'd already incurred thousands of dollars of medical costs I couldn't afford.

My father tried to insist that Prudential take responsibility; they would not.

At a time when medical treatment could still help me learn how to walk again, and maximize my usable vision, the Fates had cut off my hopes for answers and the future with a clean "snip." Self-destructive depression relentlessly crept up, a smothering sense of loss of control over my destiny, as the Fates laughed at my efforts, my time run out.

Along with the depression that accompanied the sudden cutoff of all therapy was a fatigue that took the form of long sleeping binges. The pattern repeated periodically, and I gave the shorter name of "crash" to these episodes. Though no one could tell me if I was right, I fervently hoped the crashes were a symptom of brain recovery, not to be feared, but gently worked through, just as babies fuss and complain, then sleep, as their bodies and minds grow. I always felt better after a crash, and fifteen hours or more of deepest sleep.

After desperate pleas by my parents, a representative at our local Social Security office activated Medicare coverage, but the earliest she could make it happen, the kind government official explained, was February 1 of the next year. Until then, I was uninsured and uninsurable.

I wondered what else we were told and relied upon that might be false, what other steps to full recovery the false prophets might have hidden from me. It never occurred to me before to investigate for myself. I believe all Dr. Klapper's hardware removal, Master Kim's intense physical therapy, and cognitive training with Lois began to help my brain to thread thoughts together in new ways; to synthesize them into a plan.

I remembered when O.J. Simpson's trial began that I was an attorney; now I could integrate additional facts, how I passed the California Bar at age twenty-two, the youngest in a very long time. Why not, my mind pressed, turn on my office computer, dormant nearly six years, and search the Internet? Another idea occurred to me. We called the office of our local Congressman, where a helpful aide explained some of the laws that applied, including HIPAA and a special law in California's Insurance Code, that a person whose spouse died in a disabling accident was entitled to one extra year of health coverage, for no premium. It seemed that in the business of caring, too, no one tells you everything.

Once my family discovered how to request my rights under this law, Great West reopened its extinct Music Center employee group, and granted one more year of coverage for every treatment, so long as it was for my disabling condition.

The additional year had already started to run, which gave me until the end of the following September, another ten months of full, free insurance coverage, to find my answers. It made me terribly aware of time, how every possibility for recovery depended on it.

I spent New Year's Eve at home with my parents, as celebrations of the approach of 2000 traveled around the planet. The Romans named the month of January for their god of gates and doors. An ancient Italian god of new beginnings, Janus was usually represented with two faces, one to consider what is behind, while the other looks toward all that lies ahead. In heart and mind, we're still the same people as the Romans, and the forgotten tribes who came before, whose beliefs the Romans inherited; for as a new century opened, I too faced my past, and future.

I asked myself if the extra time would be enough, and knew that no one could tell me. I wondered if Lois was right when she promised to physically block my driveway if I tried to go to Rancho for tendon transfer surgery; or Dr. Klapper, who recommended me to go there; or Dr. Banning, who advised to leave the mystery in my pelvis to the "tincture of time." It was the same maddening uncertainty, it seemed, with every question that mattered most to my health and future. After the false prophets, three things alone were certain. For the first time in my life I now had Medicare, not for reaching the age of sixty-five, but because of my disability; second, in spite of those false prophets, insurance coverage, for all my specialized treatments that Medicare didn't cover, would last ten more precious months; and third, more than ever it, was a race against time to find the hidden path.

CHAPTER FOURTEEN

WESTERN AND EASTERN RECOVERY

*Countless questions in search of an answer,
but in the end, isn't it always the same question . . . and always the same answer?*
—Narrator, *Run Lola Run*

It was all very well to watch others celebrate the millennium and make long-term resolutions for it, but to
do that myself I needed to know if I was trapped on a
recovery plateau—and if so, find the path off it as soon
as possible. Maybe, I fretted, my hidden path was nothing but an illusion. When a desperately thirsty traveler
crosses a desert and sees the mirage of an oasis, it seems
to grow bigger and bigger the closer he gets. The oasis is
huge, almost touches the sky by the time he reaches it,
when it vanishes.

Similarly, the promise of Dr. Stewart's surgery to
remove the skull hardware loomed ever larger during my
long wait for it. And although the elephant on my head

was now gone, the solution apparently reached, something inside still felt very wrong, as if I was no nearer my answer. I was on newer, even stronger prescriptions to combat Dracula eye. If repeated surgical stripping and disinfection of my jaw, and Stewart's removal of the hardware and direct application of antibiotics inside my skull, hadn't worked other than to slow Dracula down for a few weeks, I asked myself what chance I had with anything else.

So at the start of 2000, I sat in the clinic waiting room of Dr. Shangyou Zhong, the Chinese doctor Robert Klapper recommended for acupuncture and other treatments. Perhaps Robert saw my fear and exhaustion, I reflected, when I asked whether there were any choices other than a cowboy surgeon, or to dice and splice tendons in my foot, ankle, and leg. This was the one practitioner he recommended for treatment, a Chinese doctor with Western training, and as soon as my first consultation began, she and her assistant Beth made me completely at ease.

Whereas Dr. Polk focused exclusively on the site of his tendon transfer surgeries, Dr. Zhong's clinical examination addressed my body as a whole. She examined my abdomen and its many scars, identified one of my debilitating symptoms before I so much as mentioned my digestion. It was an intermittent symptom doctors were unable either to diagnose or treat, let alone cure: a sporadic, uncontrollable need for the bathroom.

Dr. Zhong immediately recommended a specific formulation of herbal tea to get rid of toxins, based on the belief in Chinese medicine that crystals form deep inside the body along with scars. I guessed it would also be true of my brain—that must be full of crystals too. If I could cleanse my circulation of scars and crystals, maybe it would help restore function.

That first day, she started me also on a regime

of Chinese medicine: acupuncture, moxibustion (which involved the heating of the acupuncture point with a smoldering herb), acupressure (or deep massage of key nervous points), and glass ampoules that were heated and placed on my body, so as the air cooled and contracted they drew my flesh up into them. Where Western medicine focuses by organ, Eastern sees one circulation, a network of systems through the body with meridians, which provide access points to restore balance by "opening the channels."

Western research supports the Eastern belief that acupuncture has specific biological effects. In a SPECT scan that viewed the brain during acupuncture treatment, scientists saw blood flow increase in a relay station for pain messages and other sensory information, as well as changes in the cortex and brain stem. The changes don't show how acupuncture works, but the fact physiological changes occur even in patients without symptoms, the control group, indicates the effects are real.

As my acupuncture session began, I watched Dr. Zhong run a wire from one needle to the next, insert them along chosen pathways, my meridians, then a little machine played a series of electronic notes, like a child's nursery rhyme.

Tum, tee, tee, tee, tum went its little overture, and current began to pass through the small wire, down the needles, into and along my nerves, stimulating them directly. There's no way to know which modality or combination of them she used was the cause—Eastern medicine is based on the principle that it's impossible to separate the components that make our bodies one indivisible whole—but my dreams grew incredibly clear and strong.

Like Shakespeare wrote, "we are such stuff as dreams are made on," and when I woke in the morning after my first session, I could still remember the vivid details of that *stuff* crystal-clear; how I dreamt in concepts of images, not the images themselves, how I looked at words written on documents in my dreamscape, and saw the language they were written in. I could remember dreams like a tape that replayed in sequence. Except, just like the whale's repeated call through the ocean, there was the smallest variation of the song every so often as my brain advanced the tape in search of linked image-concepts.

The experience made me optimistic that steady application of Chinese medicine to my body would help, and I'd go for acupuncture three times a week for the next six months. "Good for Chi!" Dr. Zhong and her clinicians often exclaimed as they worked, and felt *qi*, my energy flow, respond to their touch. Their different modalities, and entirely different beliefs, opened my mind to the possibility that maybe, if I built the right paths and opened the right doors, the nerves and their precious signals could come through. I often sensed them open in the evening after a day of Chinese therapy, when I felt nerve pulses ripple suddenly down both legs. "Warm fireworks," I called them. Sometimes, after sessions deep-stimulated my nerves and released the fireworks, I felt that to walk was maybe a question of faith; that I must stretch a foot that I couldn't feel or see out in front of me, and trust my mind knew where my body was, knew where my feet needed to be, like in *Indiana Jones and the Last Crusade* where, to pass his final test, Jones must step into an apparent abyss, when he can't see the bridge across. But by next day the warm fireworks would be gone, the doors closed again.

I had to explore East and West, and advance as fast as I could before September 30. I couldn't afford to wait for results to flow, but instead had to search for the path in other ways at the same time, even as the level and intensity of treatment rose. So with Dr. Zhong's Eastern program in place, Lois was ready with her next suggestion—a doctor with some of the most advanced medicine in the western United States.

"Drake will run all the neurology tests you need, and evaluate you for Botox," she offered. Apart from its use to release face wrinkles, administration of this dilute toxin, Lois explained, could temporarily force any muscle to relax. To prepare for three full days at this expert doctor's clinic, my internist drew five vials of blood to run all the panels required, plus body fluids to assess my neurotransmitter system, all of which we shipped with my contradictory medical opinions.

Dr. Drake Duane was the director of the Arizona Dystonia Institute in Scottsdale, Arizona, and later that month my mother and I took off from Burbank, the same route I flew so often to Marcy's hometown. As our plane descended over familiar landmarks, I saw Camelback Mountain with trails Marcy and I hiked together, and when I entered the airport lobby with its huge cactus sculptures, they confronted me with ghosts from my past that I wasn't brave enough, or ready, to face. I missed her too deeply, and knew it would lead me to a place of despair from which I'd not return.

The sessions at the Institute were intensive, and started with a brain MRI. Cedars, it turned out, never took one.

"It's always done first with head traumas," the radiology tech at a Scottsdale hospital remarked, "unless the patient's unable to comply."

My first brain MRI showed extensive scar tissue across a broad swath of my right hemisphere.

"At least it wasn't your left," the friendly tech encouraged. "You know what we say about the left brain? Never leave home without it!"

Dozens of tests followed. Sensors were glued onto my skull and EEG traces were taken as I responded to light. Computer simulations analyzed my logic circuits, literally, and there was another EMG with pins stuck in my nerves, as at Cedars and Rancho. At the end of the last day, Drake met my mother and me in his office, with my father on conference call from L.A. He described how, unlike diseases, which have common pathologies, brain injuries are as unique as each of our brains.

"In your case, Mr. Lewis, I found a pause in the transmission of signals."

He didn't sound optimistic, his tone that of a dispassionate research scientist with results from his latest experiment.

"Nerves are like railroad tracks, with a train on them to carry messages from your brain. But somewhere along those tracks—we don't know where—the train carrying information through you . . . pauses."

He recommended against tendon transfers, and against Botox injections, a therapy he frequently administered. He spoke candidly as the sun set, the shadows of the giant saguaro cactus lengthened across the desert outside his window, and his consultation drew to a close.

"Simon, I think at least three different nerve pathologies cause your dystonia—your excessive tone. Which means if I reduce that symptom with Botox injections your left leg may collapse completely."

If my body was one complete system like my Chinese doctor believed, I wondered whether regular Botox injections might, over time, spread through it.

"That's a risk," he agreed.

He offered to write a prescription for depression and made other recommendations, such as a daily dose of one type of choline—a natural dietary supplement useful to help my memory, and which I've taken ever since—but he could not offer a solution for my damaged nerves. I thought about that unknown on the plane back to L.A., about my mind's inability to regain control of my body.

"Perhaps it's the scars, Robert," I said when I went to ask him.

"It's certainly possible," Dr. Klapper agreed, with his frank open-mindedness that encouraged me. Doctors call them gross incisions, and the ICU at Cedars had made a bunch of them on admission when they checked the status of my vital organs. Perhaps my scars physically held me down.

"Is there someone you recommend to take a look?"

The best, it seemed, knew the best, because he hardly hesitated.

"I know a good plastic surgeon—go see Andy."

Dr. Andrew Berman's offices were next door to the Academy of Motion Picture Arts and Sciences in Beverly Hills, the organization that awards the Oscars. Many of Dr. Berman's patients were doubtless members; one of many plaques revealed his father was head of the American Academy of Facial Plastics and Reconstructive Surgery. He shortly appeared in person, a really cool young doctor who rushed eagerly into the waiting room to shake my hand, and from that moment I called him Andy, never "Dr. Berman."

It didn't take him long to recommend a "Z-plasty" for my abdominal scar, and at the same time he could take care of my facial scars, which was good news.

When I left, I booked my outpatient surgery at his clinic across the hall, and later was happy with the results of it, my scars greatly diminished. But Andy was a rare surgeon, and special guide on my journey, because he offered a postoperative suggestion outside his specialty to help with my recovery.

"Ever had hyperbaric oxygen?" he asked with a knowing smile. "It's often recommended for brain injury."

With over a third of my right brain gone, a recovery chamber sounded like a really good idea.

"Do you think it's too late—so long after the crash?" I wondered.

"Don't think anyone knows," Andy shrugged. "It won't hurt, and it will help your skin to heal."

By now, I was accustomed to just how little anybody knew for certain about the brain's potential; how the thing that matters most to our lives is the part of us doctors still understand the least. And despite their apparent usefulness to heal trauma victims, there were astonishingly few hospitals in L.A. equipped with hyperbaric chambers, so days later I signed into an outpatient facility in Culver City.

"Are you claustrophobic?" Connie, my nurse, asked after I changed into a cotton gown—oxygen is highly flammable, and static buildup in an artificial fabric could spark a fireball.

I didn't think I was claustrophobic from my experience in the MRI tunnel, but then I was never loaded into what looked like a clear acrylic torpedo tube, sealed at both ends with heavy reinforced doors.

"I, um, don't think so Connie . . . ," my voice quavered.

"It's nothing, really," came from the other side of the room.

"Hi, I'm Lloyd!" the muffled voice continued. Lloyd was a record producer, in treatment for throat cancer, which went into remission when he started hyperbaric oxygen. He was already loaded into the matching tube on the other side of the room, and seemed quite relaxed as the equipment hummed, and built pressure inside.

"Thanks, Lloyd!" I called back. "I'm ready," I told

Connie, and with that she slid my pallet into the long cylinder, and closed and sealed the airlock door inches above my head.

I recognized the sound almost immediately: a low hiss, as cylinder valves opened and oxygen flowed into my pod. It was from my comascape, that sound. Far down the slope of consciousness, my mind absorbed this sound, which was my constant companion for days that became weeks. I felt instantly, spiritually, at home inside my torpedo tube. As it was my first "dive" they took me down slowly, like in a submarine, and once at full pressure, they ran a video of *The Little Mermaid* for my super-oxygenated trip "under the sea." All in all, my first dive felt good.

Next morning, I headed into the bathroom to wash, and looked in the mirror at the worst Dracula eye I ever saw. Every imaginable shade of purple and scarlet, and some I couldn't imagine, suffused my eyes. When it resurfaced after Stewart removed my skull hardware, I wondered how an infection alive on my head plates could survive even their removal, and concluded it was invulnerable.

My eyes never looked this bad before, yet I never felt better about them, or more certain Dracula was dead. Somehow, I knew this orgiastic display was the last toxic release, knew the supercharged oxygen in my blood had dispelled the final vestiges of infection, wherever they lurked. Like those microbes on the U.S. flag on the moon, on some remote titanium fragment or bone spur in my skull, outside my blood and spinal fluid and invisible to scans, colonies of the Dracula bug had found a niche to cling to. And as supercharged oxygen, highly toxic to most microorganisms, penetrated the cells of my body, it reached and drove a stake through the heart of every one.

I never saw Dracula again.

I didn't understand why no one recommended this simple cure, instead dispensed palliative eye drops that gave the shortest relief, and looked forward to my next dive. I could feel the surge, the oxygen build in my blood circulation as I watched another movie play through the walls of my torpedo tube. *Ssssss*. The oxygen seemed to lift my spirits, fill me with hope.

Perhaps the oxygen helped as well in my sessions with Lois, because I made steady progress as the new century advanced. I told her how outside my hospital door at Cedars looked as if it existed in another dimension. . . . That I knew objects and people were real, but ceased to be real to me, as if outside my world. Lois totally understood, and there were many elements to her program to rebuild and integrate each facet. There were written exercises that integrated the sequencing of vision with sound and words; I drew shapes on a sheet of paper, and said the direction of each line as I drew it, in rhythm to a metronome. It was incredibly tiring.

"Over, up, down," I recited as I listened to the beat, thought about the direction my pencil traveled on the paper, and with my eyes timed its movements to the steady *tick . . . tick . . . tick . . .* of the metronome.

Little peaks appeared across the page.

"Over, up, over, down," and there was a row of crenellated battlements like a castle wall; another series created teeth. Lois gave me small wooden building blocks from Scandinavia for a grasp of shapes, sequencing, and forming strategies; "Magic Eye" three-dimensional images to help me grasp depth, and process peripheral vision; Mozart piano concertos 21 and 23 to let the music sing in my ears, shape, and expand that separate part of the brain while I worked.

And always back to Culver City, for my next refreshing hyperbaric dive. I told Andy Berman at our next appointment how much the oxygen helped, and while

I still had this great specialist's attention, seized the precious opportunity to try and continue my recovery—with a necessary step. I explained about my dentist, who said my teeth looked "fine" on top, but prescribed root canals from beneath, and about Doctor Red Dots who thought the surface of my teeth needed multiple fillings, when it was my jaw that felt wrong.

"Is there anyone you know, Andy?"

It sounded odd to ask a plastic surgeon to recommend a dentist, but with Andy's proven interest in recovery, I hoped for another great postoperative idea.

"Sure do," he grinned. "Bit into a burger once and chipped a tooth! Checked every surgeon in L.A." He paused. "I mean, I *really checked*. Barry's the man to see."

While I waited on insurance authorization for a consultation with Dr. Barry Skaggs, I felt like I'd made real progress. On my last hyperbaric dive, Connie said she was about to move on herself, to become a nurse on a cruise ship.

"There are no good men left in L.A.," she sighed as she bid me farewell. "I know, I've tried. I'm going to sail the seven seas to look for better!"

I felt hopeful when I arrived at Barry Skaggs's clinic, even if he worked in a medical specialty I never heard of, called maxillofacial surgery. According to the wall plaque in his waiting room, he was a certified diplomate of it, which had to be good, whatever *it* was. Andy Berman had mentioned Dr. Skaggs was a keen surfer on the waves virtually every day at 6:00 AM before his clinic, and as he strode into my cubicle, he certainly looked the part: athletic, blond, and very tan. It took about fifteen minutes for him to take X-rays, no different, it appeared, than the images taken by my dentist and Doctor Red Dots. But his diagnosis was totally different: infection, and extensive bone loss that required immediate surgery with a graft of healthy bone, to save my jaw.

It seemed there was no end to the threats to my body, my health, and my life that doctors misdiagnosed, or missed altogether. It was both a relief and a shock to discover this latest one. In May, when my brother Jonathan and his wife Elinor welcomed their first baby, Samuel, at Cedars-Sinai, I wondered whether I could find the same one day, to be capable not only to live independently and well enough to look after myself, but to share responsibility for the needs of a family. I was desperate to find a way forward with my own life, but could not bring myself to choose between the three different recommendations of how to cut and transfer my tendons in order to walk again, or figure out how to stop my unrelenting fatigue and headaches.

"What chance do I really have?" I asked Lois in my next session at her clinic. The temporary loss of insurance to see her reinforced just how special and helpful her therapy was; hers was the opinion I valued most on what to do next.

"How can specialists be in such complete disagreement?" I asked.

"Because our knowledge is growing fast, but no one understands the nerves—or our brains," she replied softly.

It was a quiet revelation. I remembered Dr. Whitney at Cedars, head of my rehab there, who wrote down my questions, but gave so few answers.

"Most doctors don't understand brain injury well unless they specialize in it," she went on. "So many of them are unaware of all the improvement possible, since they learned in medical school that there's none after the first year. I'm in this for the long run Simon, until completion: until I get you back to *your normal.*"

Lois understood the brain's true potential. Her goal wasn't that I passively accept whatever I had, and be grateful for it, the Harvard doctor's advice, nor that I learn how to cross a road at functional speed, the short-term goal of many physical therapists. Lois wanted me to cross something entirely different: first, the line from below average, to average; from there, to above average; and finally, cross over a special finishing line, to full cognitive recovery. But she couldn't advise me on my periodic mental crashes, nor which tendon surgery I should undergo to walk again.

Maybe I missed something, took a wrong turn to reach this dead end, but I didn't know what more I could do as September arrived, and I faced the imminent loss of insurance for most of my therapies in four weeks. It seemed a question without an answer. I remembered a story I read as a kid, of a man on his hands and knees under a lamppost late on a very dark night. He searches intently all around him in the dim pool of light.

"What are you doing?" a passerby inquires.

"I live across the street, and dropped my key opening the front door," the searcher replies.

"But your key's on the *other* side of the street by your door," the passerby queries. "Why aren't you looking over there?"

"Oh no," the first man confidently replies. "It's far too dark over there—I'd never see it!"

I felt a bit like that man, if anything worse off. He at least knew all the facts, and knew there *was* a key.

I thought a lot about that story. I wasn't even sure any more which side of the street I was on, whether I was looking in the right place, or, like that man, spent my last precious months of insurance on a search in the only light I could find, rather than where the key was. No matter how dark and futile it seemed, with only days of insurance left, I'd no choice but to keep searching for that key and hope it existed. Perhaps the greatest benefit of all the acupuncture, acupressure, and Chinese herbal tea, of the uncompromising rigor of Tae Kwon Do's exercises and philosophy, and of learning how to think again in my ongoing sessions with Lois, was a mind strong enough to find these questions and face such total uncertainty.

A mind that, at last, was capable to make some kind of plan for when September would end, and my California insurance extension run out.

For whatever lay ahead in the dark.

CHAPTER FIFTEEN

HARRISON FORD

When you wish upon a star
Makes no difference who you are
Anything your heart desires
Will come to you
> —Jiminy Cricket,
> "When You Wish upon a Star"

There was only one appointment left under my expiring insurance—with Barry Skaggs. Dr. Skaggs, the second surgeon to strip diseased bone from my jaw, hinted at the last follow-up it was essential for me to see a dentist. I must make progress on whatever front I could, I reflected in the car with my mother on the way to his clinic, as my focus shifted to my imminent appointment and greatest area of indecision and delay: my teeth and jaw.

It felt right to leave my old dentist after the unsuccessful root canals, but I began to doubt my decision to reject the enthusiastic young one in the San Fernando Valley with his X-ray, and all the fillings I needed neatly marked with little red dots. Perhaps I made my dental problems a lot worse when I delayed his work on my decayed teeth for so long. My ignorance after a lifetime of dentists, I realized, was near total. When it came down to it, there seemed no way to judge one from the next. You closed your eyes, opened your mouth while they worked their craft, and hoped for a reprieve until next time.

The only certainty was that I urgently needed a second opinion on Doctor Red Dot's fifteen or twenty fillings, and to figure out how to get sent to the best. I needed to find that lost key in the dark, at least for my jaw. Since Barry was a top oral surgeon, he had that key all right, but as dentistry wasn't his field, I needed to figure out the right question to ask him. My thoughts turned frantic as my mother pulled our car into the medical building. No doubt about it—thanks to my surgeons, doctors, and Lois Provda, under pressure my mind could speed up.

Dr. Skaggs checked his fresh X-rays. There was, he said, no sign of infection. That was a relief, but I knew what would follow.

"Do you have a dentist, Simon?"

If I said yes, I'd become the patient of Doctor Red Dots with his ready drill. Another dentist already responsible for my treatment meant no referral, no recommendation to another one, by Dr. Skaggs.

"Well, ye—," my mother began.

"No! Dr. Skaggs, I don't," I interrupted.

All my desperate thoughts came together to fill the sudden silence.

"Tell me, Barry . . . if Harrison Ford chipped his teeth, who would he see?"

This was L.A., home to the stars, with dentists

who tend the most perfect teeth in the world. I didn't know Harrison Ford, but I'd thought again about that scene in *The Last Crusade*: Indiana Jones stepping into the void. In the best tradition of American football, it was a fourth-quarter, fourth down, Hail Mary pass.

"And I'd have to go immediately," I added, "because my Great-West insurance ends in a few days," the redundant added to the preposterous.

He didn't say anything. I could see the ball of my Hail Mary pass, as it spiraled through thin air, and heard my mother's groan. But my eyes were fixed on Barry, and he didn't seem to have heard her.

"Wait here," he said, and then left.

Dr. Skaggs's receptionist arrived a few minutes later.

"I've come to take you upstairs," was all she said. It seemed a bit mysterious.

"Where are we going?" I whispered as she escorted us to the elevator.

"Dr. McKay," she offered as she held the elevator door.

"Do you think he's good?" my mother asked, on the theory that nurses know the most. Mary paused, with her finger on the button to the top floor.

"They call him the 'Leonardo da Vinci' of dentists," she said. Then she released the door, and the elevator whisked us up.

We entered a penthouse clinic where two receptionists greeted us, Laurie and Beverly. New Age music filled the air and there were bowls of fresh cut flowers.

Barry had called ahead, and Dr. Duane McKay, a man in his early forties with remarkably clear eyes and an engaging smile, emerged soon after. We thanked him several times for the immediate consultation—outside of the emergency room, no doctor had ever done such a thing. As I told him my clinical history, he summarized it into a handheld recorder.

Twice, Dr. McKay made a mistake. I described where my jaw was fractured, and pointed to the spot on the right side where hardware was implanted then removed. Except Dr. McKay, as he dictated his clinical impressions, described my "*left* side fracture."

"I'm so very sorry," he apologized the second time he made the same error, and asked us to send to his office all my hospital records. We explained how many there were, how little time was left on my insurance to check them. It seemed too much to ask of any doctor.

"Then bring your records and we'll review them together—first thing tomorrow morning!" Dr. McKay exclaimed.

He smiled brightly, with those twinkling eyes. And that was when I understood what the receptionist meant by Leonardo da Vinci, among the most prolific geniuses of history, both scientist and artist. I'd no idea what Dr. McKay was up to, as he pored over my hospital reports for confirmation of what he saw in his appraisal of my face.

"Bingo!" he exclaimed at last, with quiet satisfaction.

There it was, a report from Cedars-Sinai of a scan two days after the crash, but never followed up. It described multiple skull fractures, and Dr. McKay had zeroed in on one that indicated my jaw was out of alignment by three to four millimeters, unseen and untreated by my specialists ever since. Over the next few days, he made a full analysis of my craniomandibular system—my head and jaw—using new imaging methodologies, including a joint vibration analysis and a three-dimensional cone beam CT. Dr. McKay was one of the few practitioners in North America to integrate biomechanics and computer-enhanced graphics this way, his preliminary diagnosis as incisive as his technology.

"If you do nothing, Simon," Dr. McKay offered, "considering the nature and extent of your injuries the alignment of your teeth, muscles, and jaw joints will likely deteriorate further, until functions are compromised."

Ever since Dr. Anderson unwired my jaw at Cedars, I'd thought that part of me was saved; I had once again taken it for granted. It was hard to hear this new threat.

"Yes," Dr. McKay sighed, "I'm afraid some patients' ability to chew becomes quite limited, causing them to eat primarily soft foods. Many older people who aren't diagnosed and treated are confronted with such consequences."

In my case, he said, the jaw was broken different ways, and in different directions, on both sides. Dr. McKay couldn't change the fact that my jaw and skull were crushed. The mal-alignments, created as my fractures healed, would remain. But he believed that with careful assessment and treatment, he might manage my head and neck systems to maintain function. Guided by his computer images and past experience, he would try to change the orthopedic relationships of my upper and lower jaw, with something called an intra-oral orthotic.

"With the assistance of additional therapies," Dr. McKay added, "the orthotic should guide your mandible into a new adapted position."

"Is that better for me?" I struggled to understand.

"Yes, Simon," he smiled to encourage me, "because an adapted functional position—if we achieve one for you—would integrate and balance your muscles, teeth, and joints."

His initial evaluation was covered within the final days of my ten-month insurance extension, but I still confronted the void I was stepping into; of how to pay for the very prolonged orthodontic treatment needed to rescue my jaw.

Unnoticed, the business of caring arrived at the time of year when health insurers announce their plans for the following year. Two days after Dr. McKay's recommendation, there was a letter in the mail from the Writers Guild of America, of which I was still a member. Throughout, my mother continued all my film industry guild memberships as part of her usual maintenance of my office. It helped to keep hope alive that one day I might recover enough to return to my career.

The Writers Guild newsletter included announcement of new medical insurance—WritersCare—for all members whose Guild coverage had lapsed, so long as they were recently insured in any other group plan. WritersCare would be run by Health Net, one of America's biggest carriers.

There was, the newsletter said a short "open enrollment," the magical term that meant the insurer could not cherry-pick applicants for the brief time this door was open. It was President Clinton's HIPAA law in action, to enable people to move from one insurance group to another—health insurance portability. There was just the one huge question: of whether I qualified as a person who was "recently insured in a group plan."

I was the only member in my Great-West group. In fact, there never was anyone else after a California law forced my insurer to reinstate me in its canceled plan for a final ten months. So I was the sole insured in an otherwise nonexistent group, one with only days left to run. Would the law allow me across the threshold, onto the hidden path once more? My family rushed the completed form and first check by messenger to Health Net's offices in Woodland Hills, and waited. Almost immediately, an enrollment package arrived with my insurance identification card, for a year of coverage.

The effective start date of my WritersCare insurance was September 30, the very same date Great-West's coverage under its special extension, finally expired.

In the fall of 2000, I reached my new millennium: full health coverage, with no exclusions for preexisting conditions, for all my medical treatments.

And the Hail Mary pass is . . . completed . . . for a touchdown.

CHAPTER SIXTEEN

TURNING POINT

". . . Will you tell me where we are?" asked Tock as he looked around the desolate island.

"To be sure," said Canby; "you're on the Island of Conclusions."

"But how did we get here?" asked Milo.

"You jumped. That's the way nearly everyone gets here."

". . . I'm sure," gasped Milo. "But from now on I'm going to have a very good reason before I make up my mind about anything. You can lose too much time jumping to Conclusions."

—Norton Juster,
The Phantom Tollbooth

In the following weeks, Dr. McKay started his long-term treatment, except almost immediately Health Net wouldn't accept some of his bills; those they decided were for dental, not medical, services. I could only afford his treatment if it was covered, and my access to this stage of the hidden path was saved by another program the Cedars social workers never mentioned at the outset: the California Victims of Crime Program. There are many state and federal victim assistance programs; my mother by pure chance saw California's mentioned on TV, and we had visited their local office years before, at the Van Nuys courthouse.

It seemed a pointless exercise at the time, but my visit opened a file. Without one, my rights would have disappeared completely. With an open file, over $40,000 remained permanently available to me as the victim of a hit-and-run, from the state for otherwise uninsured medical expenses, starting with the dental aspects of Dr. McKay's restoration of my jaw.

After early success, Master Kim ramped up my ongoing sessions at his dojo, but the new level triggered worse crashes, more intense headaches, and exhaustion. I slept often for fifteen hours or more. Master Kim was concerned, and suggested yoga might help me cope. More a philosophy of life and meditation than a medical discipline, he explained, yoga might increase my balance and equilibrium, enhance awareness of my body and mind.

The next afternoon, I went to the address on Robertson Boulevard, put on my soft Tae Kwon Do shoes and sweats in the tidy changing rooms, and entered the yoga school.

What struck me was the incredible heat; it had to be a hundred degrees in there. It felt great as it sucked tension from my muscles, perhaps to make the body supple and prevent injury.

Gradually, a hundred and fifty students arrived, many of them models and actors it seemed, striving for top physical and spiritual shape. They arranged themselves throughout the room in serried rows, so as to have a good view of a low stage at the front.

I'd learned with Master Kim how to get myself down to a seated position on the floor, and waited. It felt so good to be surrounded by not only such a big assembly of motivated and interested people, but also some of the healthiest and tanned I saw in a long time. The leader of this golden group, a strikingly trim and athletic yogi, entered, sat cross-legged on the stage in one fluid movement, and achieved some graceful first postures without apparent effort.

He then started the session in a voice that resonated through the big room, with the observation that there are ten trillion cells in your body, governed by the heart, that they all vibrate at a certain frequency, and that the planet Earth vibrates with the same frequency.

"Take *mother*," the sonorous voice drifted across the assembled multitude as his sermon advanced to the next topic, his body to the next yoga position, and the class did likewise.

"Take the last four letters of 'mother'—and spell e-r-t-h. . . ."

Another move, another position, and a hundred and fifty bodies followed in unison, while the hundred and fifty-first did his best.

"Add the first and most important letter of our alphabet—an 'a'—to the middle, the center, of 'E-r-t-h' and you have our Earth," he continued gently.

"Mother and Earth are linked forever. . . ."

The insight was interesting, I thought as I struggled with the third position, except I couldn't help wonder, if yoga was an Indian philosophy, whether there was the same similarity of words in Sanskrit or French. Didn't the elemental forces of our bodies, and their relation to our planet, have to work for all nationalities and languages? For instance, almost seventy-one percent of

our planet is covered by sea, exactly the proportion of
the human body that is salt water from which our spe-
cies evolved, and that's true of every one of us, regardless of sex or national origin. Maybe we really are all
stardust, all golden.

Our leader returned to the ten trillion cells in our
body that vibrate at a frequency we all share with our
world. And when he played his gong tuned to this frequency, it imbued us with it, to heal our bodies, sharpen
our minds, and elevate our spirits.

We were heavily into the grueling program. The
yogi started some music to encourage his acolytes, and
I watched sweat pour off me onto the floor, as Indian
sitars strummed, wind instruments blew, and drums
rhythmically beat.

"Follow me, follow me . . . follow me, follow me,"
the singer's voice gently chanted the one-line mantra, as
our leader played his gong in the key of life to resonate
through, harmonize with, and presumably awaken, the
community of mind body and soul within.

Different though his approach seemed, the sincere spiritualism of yoga influenced me. The human
core that defined who I was grew beyond the physical
package I thought about in my sessions with Dr. Zhong;
it signified everything that defined both who I was and
might become. But when WritersCare denied coverage
for Master Kim's therapy and yoga, even though Dr.
Banning, my insurance-approved physiatrist, recommended him, the bill was over $6,000.

Victims of Crime agreed to a one-time payment,
but without any further insurance, I had to bow deeply
one last time, and thank Master Kim from my heart for
his insights into the calcification in my pelvis he could
feel with his hands and feet, and about which Dr. Banning and Dr. Klapper had no further suggestions.

In the first week of October, I underwent a full

"CDR"—or Continuing Disability Review—by the Social Security Administration to verify whether I was still disabled.

I couldn't sleep for several nights before. I didn't know what the rules were and no one explained them to my parents or me. I dreaded what might happen if the doctor saw I could form words and decided I no longer met their unknown requirements. On the day, a Social Security doctor watched through his clinic window as my mother drove up, saw me slowly and painfully disengage from the car, then inch into his building. He read in my records how whenever I tried either to think harder, or push harder in a physical way, it was as though I crossed an invisible line and crashed. There were six possible assessments he could make of my potential level of activity; from a top Level 1, that I was productive; down to Level 6. I was, he diagnosed after his tests, still at Level 6—a patient capable of no involvement in either organized or personal activity, whether social, educational, or vocational. Though I didn't understand the details, I knew I got the bottom grade, the worst kind of test to pass, in order to receive another three years of Medicare insurance protection.

It didn't occur to me how often I might unwittingly have jumped to Conclusions in my search for the hidden path; how much time already lost like Milo on the island in Norton Juster's *The Phantom Tollbooth*. As hard as I tried, I could see no escape from my typical state, one in which it was impossible to concentrate my mind for any length of time. My only chance was to find the cause of the crashes and cure the problem, but with every Western and Eastern modality exhausted, there was nowhere else to look.

One doctor who never jumped to conclusions was Dr. McKay. It was such an inspiration in my search for the hidden path to find a doctor whose diagnosis was so rigorous and complete.

"What's the most sensitive part of your body, Simon?" he asked at my next appointment. I'd a pretty good hunch, but was still surprised when he answered his own question.

"Your *teeth!*"

"Um, what about the palm of your hand, Dr. McKay?"

"No, if you had three grains of sand on your teeth you could tell me where each one was. You couldn't if I put three grains on your palm."

"I think I'd feel something . . . ," I began. I always enjoyed my visits to his clinic, the great insights he shared.

"Oh, you might feel something's on your palm, but not how many grains and where each is sitting. . . ."

"That's true," I admitted.

"And teeth have no nerves on the surface," he beamed. "That's what's even more remarkable. You feel where each individual grain is indirectly from the roots of your teeth up!"

It was amazing, as was the logic of his innovative approach, which wasn't to work from the visible teeth back, but from the hinge of my jaw forward; to realign the muscles, discs, and joints disrupted by my injuries into functional positions.

"And," Dr. McKay concluded triumphantly, "we've verified that your jaw's regained its stability, so we can progress to the next phase!"

Orthopedic changes he would make to my teeth biting patterns, he explained, would also modify my gums, ligaments, and supporting bone in an attempt to accommodate my jaw to its multiple fractures and displacements.

When Health Net again denied coverage for this phase of treatment as excluded dental services, the

State Victims of Crime program came through, and approved the costs.

Under Dr. McKay's supervision, his dental assistant Joanna ran computer tests and analyses, while his technical assistant Rudy took X-rays and images of the joint. The evaluation process felt like an initiation to prepare me for the treatment challenges ahead, as ABBA played on the clinic speakers,

> *If you change your mind,*
> > *I'm the first in line*
> *Honey I'm still free*
> *Take a chance on me*
> *If you need me, let me know,*
> > *gonna be around*
> *If you've got no place to go,*
> > *if you're feeling down . . .*

His team made me feel like a hopeful kid. But unlike Dr. McKay's objective precision with joint vibration analysis, jaw tracking, and tomography of my jaw, so much of the evaluations and treatment I explored seemed built on wishful hope as much as hard science. No matter what I tried, fatigue and crashes overwhelmed me. Even as I plugged away doggedly with my home exercise programs, my days didn't grow, my fatigue didn't change. It was a mental and physical disability that therapy didn't solve, and inconclusive tests seemed unable to find. I still didn't know, in my childhood story of the man who searched at night for his lost door key, whether or not the key existed. The only certainty was that if I couldn't cure my crashes, fatigue, or inability to walk, I couldn't advance any further along the path of recovery.

Guided missiles use their mistakes, which they correct repeatedly, to arrive on target. I wasn't aware of mine, so no matter how much I thought about it, I didn't know how to correct course. After my regular cognitive therapy session with Lois, I talked about what was on my mind, and she invited my mother and me to join her for lunch.

"I don't see what more I can do," I began. "There's no more surgery, and I still can't walk . . . ," I continued with sad resignation, with no more doctors for me to ask.

"Lois, I guess I'm done," I finished.

That was my inevitable and reasonable conclusion.

"Moreland's the man to see," Lois shot back. "He's the best hip doctor in L.A. See what he thinks."

My jump to the conclusion I was done with surgery, I realized, cut off further investigation. Maybe it was nothing, or maybe an overlooked key to a new door, so I seized on Lois's suggestion. With this Dr. Moreland, I was determined to know why I hurt, why I couldn't walk. Dr. Moreland, Lois said, had an entire office team in Santa Monica dedicated to hip diagnosis and replacement.

When I called, I didn't speak to Dr. Moreland, but his nurse receptionist. The conversation started well, as Nancy sympathetically listened to my case history. Even the short version took time.

"So something inside stops me from walking," I finished.

Then she asked the only question that would matter to a leading hip specialist.

"Do your hips trouble you, Mr. Lewis?"

"Um, w-well, it's more my pelvis I think," I stammered.

I knew from her sudden change of tone what was next.

"Ah, in that case Dr. Moreland can't help you."

I couldn't think of anything to say. A final ray of hope extinguished faster than I could imagine, I clung to the handset, unable to say another word, or end the connection with my last lead. The call proved two things again: that the best run with the best, and that nurses know who they are.

"You know what?" Nancy began, to break the mute resignation of a patient in despair. "You know what I'd do if—God forbid—my pelvis was broken?"

"What would you do?" I whispered from stress.

"I'd see Eric Johnson at UCLA. He's *Doctor Pelvis*, that's his thing."

I wanted to reach down the phone line and hug her.

My father, on one of his regular walks with another neighbor, Dr. Hershman, who practiced at UCLA, made a point to ask.

"Oh, Johnson's your man all right," our doctor-neighbor replied. "He treated my son when he fractured his pelvis a few years back in a climbing accident."

It was also a turning point on the path because Johnson would take me away from Cedars, where all my surgeons practiced, and into UCLA Medical Center, the other major hospital on L.A.'s Westside. We explained my case to our new customer representative at Health Net's WritersCare program, who quickly approved this consultation at a different hospital by a new doctor.

"Hi," I began on the phone to Dr. Johnson's receptionist, "I was referred to you by Dr. Moreland's office."

At the name of the doctor I never met or spoke to, the nurse immediately gave me the first available appointment to take X-ray images of my pelvis, and for me to see Dr. Johnson in early October. I felt more encouraged when I arrived at his clinic. On the reception counter lay his business card, with an embossed pelvis on it; Doctor Pelvis, just like the nurse said. I'd found the right doctor, whose existence no one, before Nancy, mentioned.

There were the usual steps. Big waiting room for the big wait, little one to wait a little more. In came an intern—the familiar doctor-in-training under Johnson—to mount the X-rays and check them. He gave it his best shot; said he saw nothing significant, and then conducted some standard tests.

"Close your eyes, and touch your finger to your nose."

Dr. Johnson entered, a striking, dark-haired surgeon in his late thirties. A man of few words, he said nothing when the intern briefly reported his findings—or lack of them—and fell silent, an acolyte in the presence of the grand priest.

He looked at the X-ray on his light board for about five seconds.

"What's *that*?" Dr. Johnson asked rhetorically.

He jabbed the same place Dr. Whittaker saw "a bit of a mystery"; the same place Master Kim planted his feet and wondered what was wrong.

"Let's do a workup."

He swept around to face his intern.

"CT scan with three-dimensional reconstruction, and CT guided injection. Let's see what's there."

As Dr. Seeger, UCLA professor of radiology, supervised the CT, I realized three things. First, that Dr. Johnson saw a way forward for my pelvis; second, that I never doubted Dr. Klapper was the best until I met Johnson; and third, that I'd yet to meet a doctor I didn't like. All of them inspire confidence, or they go into research.

While I waited for the results and next consult with Dr. Johnson, I visited David Roy on the set of *Mad Song*, the film he'd offered me, but which I was unable to produce with him.

It was great to see my old friend on the set of his first movie, and look through the viewfinder at his next shot. When it was released, the *L.A. Times* would call it a "dazzling debut."

"*H . . . O . . .*," Dr. Johnson, the man of few words, pronounced when the report came back. "Heterotopic Ossification," he elaborated.

On the wall mount in his clinic, he showed me the three-dimensional reconstruction of my pelvis that a hugely powerful UCLA computer built from each slice of data in the CT scan. It was unearthly to behold this still life of the biggest bone structure in my body.

"There's always callus—extra bone—at the site of fractures," he added tersely. "But researchers have found that when there's brain injury also, the body goes into overdrive and lays down bone in different places."

I looked at my fuzzy three-dimensional anatomy colored in shades of green and covered with half-revealed, half-hidden, pockmarks. They looked like shadowy craters in a moonscape. I said nothing, because nothing I said counted.

"'Hetero' is Latin for 'other,' and 'topic' means 'places.' So 'heterotopic ossification' is bone laid down by the body in other places," Dr. Johnson offered, to fill the silence.

I was rapt as I pored over the shapes. Still silent, as he began to open up to his appreciative audience, who prayed this man might have answers.

"There's some kind of brain-bone connection that causes the overgrowth," he added.

I felt a twinge of disappointment from his tone. I could add the next words for him.

"No one knows why—or how it works."

Maybe this doctor didn't have answers for me after all, I sighed, but then Johnson pointed very precisely to the mystery area Dr. Whittaker saw in his X-ray. I couldn't see anything at first, any more than the intern.

"No, *there*," Johnson said impatiently. Then I saw it. There was something deep inside me. "It corresponds to the site of your pain and symptoms," he added. "We can go in and try to fix all three areas in one surgery."

"Could you maybe have a neurosurgeon on your team, too?" I interjected.

He sighed. I'd jumped ahead and taken it for granted that he should try all three surgeries when Dr. Johnson needed more, what lawyers call my "informed consent."

I waited for the medical mantra.

"I have to tell you, Mr. Lewis, that to operate on both front and back of your pelvis would require us to turn you over during surgery. The safer alternative is one surgery first on the back, then a second operation on the front of your pelvis."

It was the middle of October, too close for comfort to the end of the year. A second surgery might carry over into the new year; into another business of caring lottery in which I might lose coverage, and this expert's help toward full recovery. I needed to get into the OR as fast as possible.

"Please, let's do both in one."

"One more thing," Dr. Johnson added.

I wondered what extra warning there could be beyond "you might die."

"The bone's grown back since Dr. Klapper removed the hardware, which means the bone-brain injury link is still active," he enlightened. "We'll have to give you chemotherapy and radiation to try to turn off the stem cells."

I didn't like the sound of that.

"And for maximum effect, we'll administer the chemo as soon as you're conscious."

I liked the sound of that even less.

"That's fine, Doctor," I said.

Pre-op tests were easier at UCLA than Cedars— I could do them anywhere and bring the results with me—and at the end of October, I lay once again in my flimsy, feeling good because of the IV in my arm after a successful visit from Doctor You-Know-Who.

"Another informed consent was signed in-clinic," the operation report would say. In the real world, as I lay on my gurney, Johnson stood at the head of his team of three surgeons and once again explained with his admirable brevity the risks of infection, of re-operation on the same site, and of death. And with my one good hand, I scribbled a wavy line on a document held out on a clipboard which, flat on my gurney, I couldn't see and—courtesy of Feelgood—couldn't bring into focus if I could. It was a bit late for second thoughts.

Over a surgery of many hours, Dr. Johnson and his team went in the front first, flipped me like a one-hundred-and-seventy-pound flapjack, then did the back, opening the same foot-long incisions Dr. Brien made more than six years before, and Dr. Klapper after him.

My brain, still damaged, continued to lay down more bone, and what Dr. Klapper described as bone the size of a big lemon had grown again, on the front of my pelvis. "A real mess," as Dr. Johnson put it, the fresh bone was the size of his powerful fist, and encased two-thirds of my blood vessels in that critical space in my body. On the back of my pelvis, he found and removed a bridge of solid bone that my brain built between my pelvis and spine.

The moment I resurfaced, torso freshly stapled front and back, surgery residents sped me down long hospital hallways into the Radiation Unit. I knew that from the refrigerator-like cold, and two lead-lined doors I passed through to reach it. Ominously massive doors, perhaps, but I was too grateful to be alive to feel either pain or fear. I lay in a spacious laboratory, packed with electronic equipment that was monitored from a sealed control room within it. The young doctors-in-training suddenly crowded close, grabbed my bed sheet and began the magic carpet count from Cedars that I never forgot.

"One . . . two . . . three!"

Dear God, I'll split wide open, I thought. An image flashed in my mind, of two foot-long incisions fore and aft, as they neatly unzipped and my insides dropped out. This, as the three residents heaved me across onto a sheet of Formica. I felt like an almost lifeless carcass dumped onto a kitchen countertop with no cushions or sheets that might absorb radiation. It was just me, the flimsy, and the cold block I lay on for my immediate treatment.

It was freezing in there. I thought of a slab of meat in a cold locker, as I felt the metal staples across the back of my body cut into my flesh.

There were two nurses with me in the unit, I noticed hazily. They were petite, very cute, in clown costumes complete with red wigs and clown makeup. It was Halloween, and I thought of the children, the poor kids these nurses dressed for, to help them be brave so young. They comforted me too.

As Feelgood's drugs receded and I continued to gain consciousness, I became aware of radiologists behind the control room wall, more like engineers than doctors, from the sound of it. I heard them study Dr. Johnson's surgery report, discuss, measure, and map how many rads to deliver, how to aim their gun to deliver the deadly medicine to stop the uncontrolled bone growth and terminate the right cells, limiting what the Pentagon might call "collateral damage," and I called the rest of my body.

It took a long time. They had to hit several tar-
gets with exactly the right dose; a different dose onto
each. Finally, they entered the coordinates into remote
controls that swung the radiation beam generator into
place. It was huge, tons of hardware suspended from
a ceiling gantry, and pointed directly down over my
crotch.

"Lie completely still," my cute clown whispered
as she adjusted the final protective sheet of solid lead on
my chest, and slipped away. A warning alarm sounded
from the hallway outside, then silence fell in the lab as
the massive lead-lined doors slowly sealed. I was alone
under the VW-sized irradiation gun.

It was impossible not to react, not to move, when
the whole thing hummed and shook inches from my
groin, and voices called out progress reports with each
reposition and shot of radiation.

"You may have just a little nausea," a doctor reassured, as he rolled me out of the lab. "We were close
to the area that can cause some."

It hit that night and lasted my three days at
UCLA, with two private duty nurses to help me through
the night. It made me understand what true bravery is,
what many cancer patients endure on their path.

When I returned to Dr. Johnson for him to remove
the staple sutures, he'd just returned from a combined
medical conference and skiing trip in Switzerland. He
was an impressive man, no question. The extra bone he
found in the back had bridged from my spine across to
my pelvis, a false joint that made it physically impossible for my body to walk. That was gone.

"How are you since the surgery?" he asked after
discharge, at my final follow-up with him.

"It's helped a lot, but I still feel there's a problem
in the pelvis."

"I'm very sorry to hear that," he said. "With everything I found and fixed, I hoped for much more."

It was rare to hear a surgeon say that, and Dr. Johnson wasn't a surgeon to be denied satisfaction.

"Let's have a neuro check your spine," he added.

As with each specialist so far, it had worked very well to risk my life to search for the hidden path, and better yet, this newest stretch of it brought me to UCLA Medical Center. As a research hospital, UCLA had the funds to treat complicated cases and attract the best new doctors, with facilities for their research. Johnson's team had a good idea of new specialists to consult, with referral to a Dr. Stone to check my left shoulder—which still troubled me even after removal of the buckets of debris—and to Dr. Julian Flores, a spinal neurosurgeon and rising star at UCLA.

Dr. Johnson didn't want me to give up, on its own a cause for optimism, and we were assured Dr. Stone was the department's most experienced shoulder doctor. No doubt he was, but the easiest way to jump to Conclusions is courtesy of a doctor's failure to properly diagnose a medical condition.

When Dr. Stone examined my arm and shoulder in his clinic, reviewed the inconclusive EMGs, and commented, "Well, you don't have thoracic outlet syndrome," I jumped to the conclusion I didn't, with no idea what he meant when I made the jump.

Dr. Flores proved to be a thoughtful surgeon in Dr. Johnson's department, who ordered a spine MRI, carefully studied it, and could find nothing significant, specifically that there was "no Babinski's." No one could tell me whether it was a benefit from Dr. Johnson's huge surgery, but if this unhealthy symptom of my brain injury was gone, this damaged piece of my mind reassembled, maybe Lois was right, and others could heal too. As 2000 ended, I started once more to feel hope.

CHAPTER SEVENTEEN

DEUS EX MACHINA

Life is unbelievable.
Miraculous, sad . . . wonderful.
—Chorus,
Mighty Aphrodite

"If it's not my pelvis or spine, is there anything else you can do?" I asked Dr. Flores in the new year. I felt good about UCLA's rising star who recommended against spine surgery, and this was my last appointment.

"It *hurts* here—all my problems feel like they're *in here. . . .*"

I jabbed my fingers at the back of my pelvis.

Dr. Flores hesitated and there was the momentary silence I still feared and dreaded, when my recovery hung in the balance.

"Maybe it's the piriformis," he said thoughtfully. "Aaron Filler does that, I think, but you'll have a long wait."

I knew how rare it was to get a surgeon's recommendation outside his specialty, and grabbed it.

A few scribbles yielded his referral. Because it was so difficult to get an appointment, Flores promised to write a letter too.

"Dr. Filler's developed an MRI technique to image peripheral nerves," he added, "that might show why you can't walk."

My spirits rose at the thought that Dr. Filler's MRI machine might save me. The ancient Greeks invented the rules of drama we still use in movies and TV, and sometimes the writer needed a machine to finish his story. An ancient crane lowered the actors, dressed as Greek gods, to resolve all the different conflicts in the play. It makes life so much easier when someone drops out of the sky with all the answers, and Filler's machine promised just such an easy end to the hidden path I followed.

While I waited to meet Filler, Dr. Stone the shoulder man sent me for an arthrogram. Whatever the problem was with my shoulder, despite intense and increasingly gruesome efforts, two junior residents couldn't get their needle into it. It wasn't easy to listen as the two struggled with their class assignment. After they found a way in, we all stared at the inside of my shoulder on a monitor, a jumble of bone and blood vessels, while they wondered aloud to each other why the plunger was stuck and whether the needle might snap.

"Push a bit harder," the enthusiastic resident counseled, very gung ho.

"Um . . . I'm not so sure," the cautious one on the plunger replied.

"Sure you can!" the first urged, eager to break through the hidden barrier.

When Dr. Seeger, the head of musculoskeletal radiology, arrived and took control, she managed to squeeze in a tiny amount.

"It's good," she said. "All the effort was therapy for your shoulder."

Sure enough, on the way home, my arm felt the warmth of my blood, the cold of objects I touched—the most wonderful sensations I felt since the crash. They were fantastic, and lasted fifteen minutes, a clue that some barrier remained inside my shoulder. If I could feel my nerve pulse temporarily when it was dislodged, there had to be a way, in the Chinese sense, to hold the channel open.

And Dr. Stone encouraged me, because he seemed impressed I was on Filler's waiting list. It was clearly worth it, no matter how long it might take, to see my deus ex machina.

Through my mother, I'd stayed in touch with my USC film students, in particular with one graduate, Stu Pollard. On his suggestion, the graduate films screened at the end of the semester seven years ago, while I was in critical condition, were dedicated to their absent professor. After waiting patiently, Stu could at last invite me to a screening of a feature film he wrote and directed. It felt good to shake his hand, renew the friendship after so long and talk about his movie, in the belief that I was close to some answers.

Following Dr. Stone's recommendation, I booked time to see a Dr. Casper Endiman for tests of my shoulders and spine, to investigate whether the numbness and tingling in my extremities would worsen as I aged until I lost all use of fingers and hands, or if, on the brighter side, anything more could be done to hold open those nerve channels. Dr. Endiman, it appeared, performed a special procedure called a "nerve block."

Just before the appointment with him, our regular calls to Filler's receptionist paid off with an appointment days after Dr. Endiman. It was perfect: he could prepare his special images, and send them straight on to Filler.

At the initial consultation, Dr. Endiman proved a young and enthusiastic neurologist, who agreed to administer the nerve block Dr. Stone suggested, and also gave me a sample of a new drug to try that "just came in" from the manufacturer. It was a small white pill called Zanaflex, which, the little box breezily proclaimed, was "a new treatment for the management of increased muscle tone associated with spasticity."

It looked harmless enough, but that night I took half of one to be safe.

Soon, I felt strangely cozy, and grew steadily more so as I lay beneath my comforter. Waves of pure euphoria gently followed. They cradled me, and then swept me higher, ever higher, into realms of unimagined calm. Heavens above, this drug was good, and well named too, with its subtle hint of deliverance of users to Xanadu, the mystic mountain.

> *In Xanadu did Kubla Khan*
> *A stately pleasure-dome decree:*
> *Where Alph, the sacred river, ran*
> *Through caverns measureless to man*
> *Down to a sunless sea.*

Far down the slope of consciousness, a question formed and served itself up for conscious processing. It surfaced in the form of a faint nagging doubt: How I could feel so good, when I'd done nothing to deserve it? I was brought up steeped in the English tradition that the only true satisfaction was the kind you earned with effort—to be more exact, with *hardship*.

Per ardua ad astra, the motto went, like on the coat of arms of the very English family in Rider Haggard's novel, *The People of the Mist*, and adopted by several air forces since: "Through struggle to the stars."

I believed struggle was necessary for achievement, and began to feel misgivings, even as my brain savored the sweet euphoria and free associations that swept through every corridor of my mind except this one, which harbored a fragment of doubt, that this unearned bliss was too good to be true.

All too soon, my euphoria crested; the once mighty ocean swell turned in the blink of an instant into a roller coaster that fell from beneath me, and I dropped into freefall. My brain, stripped of its unnatural, unearned surge of neurotransmitters, now hungered for their replacement.

My eyes felt ready to burst out of my head, the pressure inside so great it seemed to force my brain to press hard against the rough insides of my skull. Once again, I lay and massaged my forehead, then staggered around my darkened room in the midnight hours, as the pain reached its shrieking crescendo. A crash; my Van Gogh book my solace in the moonlight until dawn.

"That's okay," Dr. Endiman said amiably, when I eventually recovered sufficiently to face whatever his test might involve, "I thought it was worth a try."

He was so enthusiastic and cheerful, which was just as well, given how painful his injections and nerve blocks were. I barely noticed his report, "Impression: normal study." All that mattered was he captured the images, and promised to forward them urgently. After my long wait, I would, at last, meet Dr. Filler. Awake and asleep, the possibility this doctor might let me walk again filled my mind.

The UCLA Department of Neurology waiting room was packed, more like an airport departure lounge, as my mother and I sat in it, anxious for my latest referral in search of an answer. Finally, a nurse called my name and I was led into Dr. Aaron Filler's office.

There was a timeworn gray metal desk from the seventies, if not earlier, with a phone and chair to match, a light panel on the wall, and an examination bench with a standard issue, clinic toilet paper cover stretched over it. There was no sense of any grand contraption lowered from the sky to save me; instead, this felt more like *The Wizard of Oz*, when Dorothy got to meet the Wizard. I prayed silently that he would be more helpful than the Wizard behind the curtain at the end of that movie.

"Good morning," Dr. Filler said as he entered and turned his attention to Endiman's nerve block images of my shoulder. "Hmm, wish I'd done these myself."

I wondered why no one in his clinic suggested that, but said nothing to the man who could have the answers I sought.

"What did you do for a living before the crash?" he asked, to distract me.

His trick worked. Too focused on my explanation, I barely noticed as he lifted my arm and took my pulse. Dr. Filler apparently decided my goals were worthwhile, that he could help me achieve them, and prescribed one of his MR neurograms. I'd get the benefit of whatever this machine could do, and felt good as we left UCLA, but that night suffered a huge crash. Doctors often asked me to rate my pain on a scale from one to ten, and I lay awake all night and wondered just how far above ten the scale could climb.

A test as advanced and expensive as a neurogram required six procedure code approvals before I received insurance authorization to lie inside the special MRI. It left a strange sense of exhaustion, as if it mildly cooked my body, and I'd more questions for my second visit with this man and his wonderful machine, but none of my symptoms or questions mattered because Dr. Filler had mounted the neurograms on his light panels and analyzed them before we arrived.

"The nervous system," he offered, "is like a garden hose filled with water. Step on it, and you get compression—less signal gets through."

Before his research, he explained, MRIs showed the spinal column, but peripheral nerves only for the first half-inch or so, before they completely disappeared from sight.

"Beyond that point, surgeons pretty much guessed where the compression was," he added. By careful adjustments to the most advanced MRI system available, Dr. Filler could capture images of those delicate, precious threads of life within us.

"Come, look!" he eagerly gestured for me to join him at the light board. It was show-and-tell time, deus ex machina time.

"There it is," he murmured reverentially.

With the point of a pencil, Dr. Filler carefully traced a faintly visible, thin gray ribbon of nerve that wound through the image.

"Right *there*, in your shoulder," he explained. "It's curved when it should be straight, because something's pressed against it."

No one before Dr. Filler so much as hinted my nerves were like compressed water hoses, and under some kind of pressure that interrupted their neural flow. And certainly no one had ever suggested that there was a way to see where this was taking place.

Rather than the piriformis diagnosis I came to him for, he would begin with four other procedures, to release the nerve entrapments he saw.

"I'll book the OR for nine hours," he added, "so I'm not in a hurry."

As I reeled from the thought of a whole day on the operating table, he followed with the mantra. Once again, my surgeon assured, I might die. As I waited, swept by waves of temptation to call it off, my family's

selfless love and support helped me face the risk of either death or disappointment.

My mother had indeed not left my side since the
crash, just as she told my father and the family around
our dining table the morning after it. My parents hadn't
taken a vacation together in seven years, and my father
really needed a break from his daily work routine in
the stock market. There was an opportunity to take an
apartment in Tel Aviv right by the sea and they asked
me to come with them, to rest before my ordeal.

"I can't!" I snapped, shaken by the idea of such
distant travel more than if I was a hundred years old.
And, I realized suddenly, I still didn't know if or how this
would ever change, still didn't know what was missing
within my head that used to make me feel like me, or
understand what blocked even this goal. I was, though,
glad my parents would get their first break.

When they left for Israel, I'd advanced to the point
I could heat frozen meals, plan my day, and watch movies, but my crisis of confidence grew as I read a letter
Dr. Stone, the shoulder expert, sent to all his patients,
explaining that because of "the managerial care situation in L.A. . . . doctors were forming a union. . . ." In
response, he planned to move to Oregon to escape California's overstressed medical system altogether.

I thought about how my recovery could continue only so long as I'd medical insurance, and how the
dim outline I first encountered at Social Security inter-
views slowly became clearer. It seemed the system en-
sured I, like millions of Americans trapped in the same
catch-22, couldn't try to make a living because I would
lose Medicare coverage to pay for further rehabilitation.
I scribbled a first hesitant note about how I might some
day write about all the people with stalled hopes and
forbidden futures.

My parents returned from Israel, and on doctor's orders I took a physical. My internist questioned whether my heart could cope with so many hours of surgery—it suffered from "sick sinus syndrome." For the first time in my life, I needed a cardiologist, and saw my father's very experienced specialist, Dr. Bersohn, who cleared me.

For my full day in the OR, I showed up well before dawn, confirmed the four parts of my body to be operated on, and soon lay, tagged and naked on a gurney in my cotton flimsy, and wondered if this surgery was my "next," or my "last"—in the bad way.

In my limited field of view was a white-coated medic, who casually walked through the supposedly secure pre-op area in one direction, then a bit later tiptoed back in the other. At first I wasn't sure it was the same guy; the second or third time I was. On this pass, he walked on exaggerated tippy toes in his blue paper booties, as if in a silent movie. Even if I was about to die—maybe especially if I was—I had to know.

"Mind if I ask what you're doing?"

He winked back conspiratorially.

"It's like this, man," he shared his secret, "the operating room never returns the pillows you guys go into surgery with. So the only way to get a-hold of some for you here in pre-op is if I dress up, slip past the nurses into the OR, and steal 'em back!"

It was hard to believe budget constraints made even this basic and essential supply scarce, or that it took this tactic for my caring intern to do his job and make patients comfortable. The name of my pillow-recycler was Tim. He checked my chart, the all-day procedures ahead, and nodded.

"Wow, good luck, dude. Gotta go!"

And with that Tim set off again. This time, he slid his feet out and leaned back like a circus clown in imaginary giant shoes, as he headed off to confound nurses with his disguise, and recycle more pillows.

Because of the length and risks of this surgery, I awoke from it in TED hose—long stockings up to the crotch—and pants that periodically inflated to prevent blood clots.

Junior members of Filler's surgical team came to visit, all smiles.

"We found pressure on your nerves *exactly* where the neurograms said we would!" one proclaimed.

"And the nerves are still intact!" said another.

They bubbled with cheer and excitement, but as night fell and I lay almost rigid on my bed, waves of drug-induced depression swept through me, punctuated by pain from the intermittent pneumatic crush on my legs. The worst was over, and I fell into my hospital night survival mode of a meditative gaze through the darkened windows until dawn. But hours later, in the dead of night, a nurse appeared.

"Come," he ordered quietly, not to disturb my neighbor in the shared room, in a thick Russian accent.

"My name is Viktor," he whispered. "Is necessary you walk!" he hissed to my second question.

He sounded impatient now, as he unplugged my inflatable pants from the breathing machine.

"But my IV . . ."

Oh no. I discovered those things could disconnect too. I was out of excuses, and Viktor was not to be denied. The instructions on my chart said patient was to get out of bed and stand up. Hospitals were forced to under staff wards and overwork their therapists, so the fact that it took Viktor until now to complete his caseload and get to me, didn't change the orders.

Like Jethro Tull sings in "Locomotive Breath": "The train, it won't stop going, no it won't slow down." Viktor and I were going on a midnight walk.

Late the next morning, a new man arrived to

share my room. Like all patients after surgery, he'd eaten nothing since his fast the night before.

"I'm starving. Where's lunch?" came his plaintive voice.

"You can eat just as soon as your stomach gurgles," the nurse insisted in a matronly tone. The shadow play behind the curtain that separated us resumed once his surgeon arrived.

"Good morning, I'm Dr. McBride," boomed a voice through the thin fabric, authoritative, and entitled to be. McBride, I knew, was Chief of Neurosurgery.

"I'm *starving*," his patient complained again. "Nurse said my stomach should be gurgling by now and I'd like some lunch!"

It reminded me of questions I so often asked myself after surgery. It was hard to think of one simpler to answer, or anyone better to ask than your nurse. McBride's incisive voice cut through the curtain.

"Forget what the nurse told you. . . ."

It sounded like heresy.

"Everyone here is a therapist, and too many people give instructions. You must only listen to me."

I thought about how I listened to Viktor, and my nightmarish midnight walk.

"If you eat now," McBride continued, "you'll go back into surgery."

The patient drew in breath to speak, but had no chance against McBride.

"Your surgery was complex. I had to go in through your stomach to get to your spine. You'll bloat for three to four days."

His patient said nothing. I was a little awed too. I never heard a doctor speak so conclusively.

"Disregard all the instructors who say you'll feel stomach action and gurgling after one to two days. You won't. *A meal right now could kill you.*"

On that happy note, McBride left my disconsolate neighbor.

Minutes later, food service placed a hot three-course lunch on his bed-tray, the meal that could kill him, and it smelled *so good!*

It was Greek tragedy and black comedy, like eternally, desperately thirsty Tantalus, who was surrounded by water he could never drink. So there lay Tantalus, famished from his fast, and much worse, because the food that could kill my neighbor was eminently reachable; it was right under his nose. When my mother arrived, she tracked down the food service staff. It was my lunch that almost killed Tantalus.

Dr. Filler came by to check on my progress, and with bad news. There was a hematoma in me, he announced, a very big one. He said the anesthesiologist added a blood thinner to the mix that Filler didn't often see in use. Maybe that's why I sprung a leak inside, which I gathered was the simpler phrase for a hematoma. Too late, I understood what McBride told his patient, and wished I heard his hospital survival speech before I met Viktor. I didn't have the heart to tell Dr. Filler about my midnight walk.

"What's to be done, Aaron?"

"Well," he pondered, "there's a risk I'll have to open you up to stop the bleeding if I try anything aggressive."

And he was gone. No more Viktor, and no physical activity of any other kind was possible. I was confined to my bed for the next two days, motionless but for the inflatable pants, until I was safely discharged home. When it came, the operation report ran eleven pages, and reported the release of all kinds of entrapment of neck and thoracic vertebrae.

Surgeons seemed to regard physical therapists as interchangeable, but this time I got lucky. I met Joyce

Wilkinson, one of UCLA's most experienced. The difference between the good, the bad, and the great therapists
is subtle, and Joyce was one of the best. At our first session, she explained the right equipment to purchase for
use at home, and when her evaluation ended before we
accomplished much, she honestly explained why.

"Sessions used to be an hour. Now they're down
to as little as twenty minutes, and fewer of them."

I'd seen it before, the signs of a system squeezed
ever tighter, the time allocated to patients for recovery shortened. But the new element that outweighed
all else came in the second session, when Joyce began
craniosacral massage therapy, and gently mobilized my
neck and skull. She explained the current research, and
her beliefs; her approach to therapy.

"The bone of your skull—it's not fixed after the end
of childhood like they used to teach. It moves," she said.

It was difficult to think clearly almost as soon as
she began, my head felt so *heavy*. "The bones in your
head move all the time, except if hardware locks it down.
And scars can do the same," she added.

After Dr. Stewart's removal of the head plates released my skull, I thought the doctors could do no more
to help it. Through the heaviness that progressively en-
veloped my mind, I hazily wondered what else might
be in there, overlooked. Joyce's massage reminded me
of sensations I felt from Chinese acupressure, and her
therapy began to turn my mind inward for answers, to
look for something that still lay *within*.

With Joyce's skill, the early results from Dr. Filler's massive surgery seemed encouraging, though my
crashes, inexplicably, continued. I was too weak on the
first follow-up at his clinic, when he removed my sutures, to do more than feel relief as he unwrapped multiple layers of bandages and dressings. As for my second
follow-up, I was by now accustomed to surgeons who

were already focused on their next surgery. Dr. Filler certainly was. As he scheduled me for the piriformis surgery, he seemed to have a comprehensive plan.

"We'll release the bands which compress your sciatic nerves, Simon," he explained, "and see what function you recover in your legs."

Encouraged, I decided to buy my first pair of trainers in a long time, and capitulated to the longstanding prescription for a leg brace, the AFO, to increase my walking endurance. I couldn't bear my immobility any longer, nor bring myself to cut and split my leg tendons. With new shoes, my brace, and a cane, I tried to walk more, to push off the plateau of my recovery, but along with sores from the AFO's hard plastic came unbelievable fatigue, accompanied by a new kind of barrier to recovery. Symptoms, hidden far down the slope of consciousness relentlessly advanced higher, to where I consciously felt them. More disabling than the pressure of the solitary elephant I felt from the head plates, these massed in numbers and intensity to climax in unharnessed stampedes through my mind. Herds of elephants that flattened all in their path—uncontrolled panic attacks.

Whereas crashes caused light sensitivity and pain in my head, there was usually neither in a panic attack. I was simply frozen in terror, as every nerve in my brain, every cell in my body, and every fiber of my being signaled doom. Ten trillion panic buttons according to my yogi as he played his gong to help soothe them with the key of life, and I felt fear in every one.

Now I understood what Dr. Croft meant at Cedars, when he defined courage as the decision each morning to "open my eyes." The attacks continued, violent, barbaric and overwhelming, until I found the will to open them, and the phantom elephants retreated. On my third follow-up with Dr. Filler at the end of the year, I came prepared with written questions, but he already reviewed a new set of neurograms from his machine, and confirmed them with a fresh nerve block by Dr. Endiman.

"The smaller surgery to help your left leg is a release of your femoral cutaneous nerve in the groin," he began, and neatly jumped across many symptoms and my questions about them.

While I coped with the thought of those further cuts into the front of my groin involved in his "smaller procedure," Dr. Filler continued.

"Your biggest issue is the nerve that's causing so much pain," he explained. "After it leaves the spine, both sciatic nerves run down your legs through a muscle—the piriformis."

I thought of Dr. Klapper and the space he described between the tail of my spine and top of my leg. It sounded like my saga could have a happy ending after all, thanks to this man's machine.

"I can resect—cut away—some of the piriformis muscle on each side so it doesn't press on the nerves," Dr. Filler continued, "then wrap it around with a special polymer, to protect the sciatic nerves while the scar forms. The polymer gets reabsorbed—and you should get real relief."

If I didn't die, which he next advised was a distinct possibility during the two surgeries.

"Which side first?" Dr. Filler asked.

It wasn't easy to choose, what with the obvious redundancy of the question if I died during the first piriformis. I struggled to focus.

"Um, can you do both sides at once?"

"Not with my operation on your femoral nerve as well. Too risky," he shook his head. "I can't move you twice."

Surgeons, it appeared, liked to go one side at a time, with the exception of Dr. Johnson with my pelvis. I opted for the left side to see if it would help free my left leg to walk, though in truth most of the pain was down my right leg.

"So, Simon, to let your body recuperate fully, perhaps we should schedule this for February?" Dr. Filler concluded.

When February came, Dr. Bersohn, now my cardiologist as well as my father's, needed to double check whether my heart could make it through Filler's second massive surgery. I was wired once more with a twenty-four-hour Holter monitor and kept a diary to record my activities. A device like a microphone assessed the sounds my heart made inside my chest and Dr. Bersohn gave the green light.

Once again, I arranged to be Filler's first case, except this Doctor Feelgood wasn't slick like last time, but inexperienced; likely a doctor-in-training. No one seemed to have told him the "oops!" rule—never to say it—or maybe he missed that class in medical school, because instead of it he said, "sorry," which was just as awful. Several times he stuck me in the wrong place.

"Hmm . . . sorry," he said yet again, then a bright afterthought struck him, "If this doesn't work, maybe I'll try to go into your left leg!"

"They're operating on the top of my left leg—femoral cutaneous nerve," I croaked.

"Oh! Sorry. . . ."

When UCLA discharged me, my mother, ever supportive, figured out how to keep the multiple bandages that swathed my whole body clean and dry. She cut the end out of a double lined large plastic garbage bag, ready for me to wear like a poncho.

In the morning, I waddled into the bathroom to wait for her, and surprised a spider in the tub. A rush of fear and depression flooded me. Almost eight years after the crash, I still was helpless as a child, and couldn't move quickly enough to catch or deal with a spider. I watched it skitter around the bathtub, its delicate legs try futilely to climb out, before inevitably it slid back down the smooth porcelain. I didn't know if I'd any better chance of escape from my condition than the spider, and unlike me, the spider was healthy. When my mother returned, it would be released and on its way.

At Dr. Filler's follow-up, I went ready once again with notes. Indeed, there was total relief of my left sciatic pain, so that part was a success.

"Yes," he said, "in places, your sciatic nerve's the size of your thumb, and the pressure on yours was so great the band made a divot in it!"

"But it's still numb," I pointed out, hesitant.

"It'll take six months just to resume its shape but it's still functional," he replied. Dr. Filler didn't seem so busy somehow and had more time to discuss my case than usual.

"The common—and wrong—approach," he continued, "is to assume there's one problem and one answer. But when there's serious trauma, we have to advance one problem at a time."

"Next step, *right* piriformis muscle, you mean?"

Dr. Filler hesitated, and then nodded.

Whatever lay beyond that step, he'd release my other sciatic nerve. But I'd got fewer answers than I hoped, when August found me once more on a surgical gurney in my cotton flimsy.

This time he had a question for me.

"How deep would you like to go?" he asked. "General or epidural?"

With an epidural, he explained, I'd be awake, and if he found he needed to go further inside, must give me even deeper shots. I recalled the two residents with their needle stuck in my shoulder, and asked myself how much I wanted to hear operating room discussion.

"You know what, Dr. Filler, every surgery so far

has turned out more complicated than expected. Ask Feelgood to take me down all the way."

A four-hour surgery followed to release and relieve not one, but as it turned out, two nerves, and I was sent home the same day. True to form, it was a bigger job than Dr. Filler foresaw from the radiographs, general anesthesia the right choice after all, and I "should get some relief," as he said the first time, so many procedures ago.

I'd noticed how surgeons typically said my condition was much worse than it looked in their images, and underestimated the time it would take to recuperate. Maybe their uncertainty about how long it would take to come back was because no one entirely understood how anesthetics worked to send you away in the first place.

It was, a nurse confided as I rested after that surgery, as much an art as a science. As to how they leave the body, my experience was that the drug didn't drop straight out next day, but somehow persisted, and instead cycled very slowly out of my system—rose and fell, but with each fall dipped lower, until its effects finally disappeared. Maybe it gradually works its way higher up the body, as it persists in the brain and central nervous system, or that's simply where I noticed it, but two areas I always felt the anesthetic make its final exit, and that I learned to look forward to, was through arm pits, and then scalp, the very top of my body.

"Will these bands come back?" I asked Dr. Filler when I returned to his clinic.

"Only a five percent chance of return," was his reply.

"Where do they come from?" I pressed. If I knew that, maybe I could prevent more in the future, but no such luck.

He shrugged. "Bands can come from scars, old blood leaks, damaged muscle fibers . . ."

"So could they be the reason for my stomach troubles?" was the final question on my list.

We were well off his medical specialty, but I still so wanted to believe in his machine. I described the symptoms: how my stomach bloated and the rush to the bathroom after meals.

"What's the answer, Dr. Filler?" This one I really needed to know.

"I suppose I might also review that and scan for attached tissue," he replied, a little distant. "But it's really hard to resolve surgically without causing bigger problems—and regular tests likely wouldn't show an intermittent mechanical problem from an injury."

In the spring, I was invited to a reception at my attorneys' Westside offices. The receptionist checked the guest list, smiled, and then handed me a blank badge to add my name and company. I tried to make small talk with Hollywood movers and shakers as they chatted, comfortably labeled as studios, TV networks, and production companies, and imagined their unspoken question of my relevance there, a disabled person with no job.

My stomach was the other reason that forced my almost immediate departure from the reception. Head injury is sometimes called a silent epidemic, because victims feel work and social pressure to hide their problems. Maybe another silent epidemic was this debilitating condition, for which I could find no diagnosis or solution. Joanna, the great dental assistant at Dr. McKay's clinic, described it after another uncontrollable need for the restroom forced my prolonged disappearance from his waiting room.

"A number of our patients seem to suffer that way after they've had abdominal surgery," she confided. To function in public I needed an explanation and cure, but could guess her answer to my question before I asked.

"No," she said. "No one knows why. . . ."

No one seemed to know what caused this symptom, but everyone had suggestions. Perhaps I ate too much fruit, too much fat, overripe fruit, fruit that wasn't ripe enough, or maybe it was the kind of milk I drank, and on and on.

I couldn't move either fast or far, yet every moment in public had to plan for emergency. In addition to my vision difficulties and sense of irrelevance, it was this problem, that my doctor could neither diagnose nor cure, which forced me to leave my friend's lavish reception almost immediately.

I began to have similar thoughts about Aaron Filler as when I neared the end of Dr. Klapper's surgeries; that if I was to figure out where the hidden path led next, I had to look for clues, like Adrian Monk or a modern Sherlock Holmes. The suspects were pretty much every part of my body and brain. My witnesses were the doctors and nurses who, just like in a detective story, often gave different answers. Except a lot of the time, I couldn't understand them—then I felt more like Inspector Clouseau.

I wasn't ready to acknowledge that I could lose confidence in either Dr. Filler or his machine. I depended on them, acutely, because after early relief, my chronic sciatic pain returned on both sides. If it got worse, I'd be confined to a wheelchair, so there was no alternative; I had to believe in him. But he seemed preoccupied at my next follow-up, and I got only one answer as he conducted his evaluation, when I told him what I'd read on the Internet.

"What's the point of an EMG," I smiled cautiously, "if they only sample a few nerves?"

"Because," Dr. Filler answered as he finished his examination of my elevated leg and healed incisions, "they tell you if there's a loss of neuron flow coming from higher up than the needle insertion point."

He shook my hand and added a last note of uncertainty.

"But the problem is, they tell you nothing about
where above the needle the loss is occurring."

October came—the business of caring time of the
year—when insurers made decisions for their new policies, and the WGA newsletter I dreaded arrived in the
mail. It said the Guild would continue its WritersCare
program—so I could breathe easy—but not with Health
Net. My choice, the newsletter advised, was to drop
out completely or transfer to the new carrier the WGA
signed onto its WritersCare program; what in England
they call "Hobson's choice." Hobson, the story goes, was
a Cambridge stable owner in the sixteenth century who
had only one horse available for hire. Yet Hobson's im-
mortal quirk was he always asked customers to "take
their choice" of which one they'd like to ride.

The WGA offered this coverage option in the very
last week of October, to be effective as of November 1.
Everyone who stayed in the WritersCare program would
transfer from Health Net to the new plan that sounded
even better. It was called UniversalCare and my primary physician at Prairie Medical Clinic would be Dr.
Thomason. It was a great take-it-or-leave-it offer that I
grabbed with relief. The business of caring test survived,
I was safe for another twelve months, and with parents
in tow, went to my last follow-up with Dr. Filler.

His office was very quiet compared to when I first
sat in his crowded waiting room, a year and a half before.

"You've released all the bands on Simon's nerves?"
my father began.

"I think so," Dr. Filler said.

"But they gave Simon only temporary relief," my
mother tried. "Is there anything else you can suggest to

help him use his leg?"

"I don't think so," he said after a pause.

My deus ex machina was a very fine surgeon and a caring man, but his apologetic tone was unmistakable. Far from a triumphal descent from the heavens to hand out all the answers like in a Greek play, the harsh reality was that Dr. Filler and his machine achieved all they could. And they hadn't enabled me to walk again.

I was, after all, worse off than the man under that streetlight. I'd searched in the wrong place for a key that didn't exist. I'd lost my last chance to find the best medical treatment, lost my way. My quest was over. I found I couldn't speak.

"And what about these terrible crashes?" my mother persisted.

I could barely hear her, her voice sounded muffled.

"Yes, Doctor," my father picked up her question urgently, worried I'd fallen silent. "Like we've kept saying, there's whole days on end my son can't get out of bed. His crashes and panic attacks—they're *worse*."

I didn't understand the point of their questions, unaware of my jump to another conclusion. Since I described my crashes to him at the outset, I assumed he factored them into his treatment plan and there was no diagnosis for them. The conclusion I jumped to was that if all his surgical procedures didn't stop my crashes, he could offer no further help. I became aware of a long silence, and began to wonder why Dr. Filler hadn't adopted an "end of consultation" voice and bid us goodbye.

His silence after my parents' desperate questions became interminable.

"Hmmm," came his hesitant voice at last. "Well . . . Dr. Saxton gets the interesting headaches. . . ."

CHAPTER EIGHTEEN

WHEN TWO AND TWO MAKE FIVE

You can't always get what you want
But if you try sometimes
*   you just might find*
You just might find
You get what you need
                    —The Rolling Stones,
       "You Can't Always Get What You Want"

Early in November, my mother and I presented my brand new UniversalCare card at the Prairie Medical clinic, and waited to meet my internist, eager for his referral to Dr. Saxton, and immediate help with my crashes. Dr. Thomason, late forties and bearded, finally joined us.

"Mr. Lewis," he said, as he cautiously extended his hand. "What are you doing here?"

It's not the first question you expect from your new primary care doctor, before he's so much as checked your pulse. It seemed safest to ignore the tone of his question—maybe it was a busy morning.

"Um, Dr. Filler—" I began nervously.

"Who is that?"

"Uh, he's my neurosurgeon at UCLA."

"And he's treating you?" There was a spark of interest.

"Yes, Doctor," I said relieved, "he's just completed surgery on me, and—"

"I can't refer you to him, but it was nice to meet you."

Polite and final, Thomason was done, and with no mention of Dr. Saxton.

"Why not?" I blurted, anything to keep him in the room.

"We've been trying to put Simon back together for almost nine years," my mother pleaded. "What's the problem?"

Dr. Thomason saw our distress. "Look," he said, "we have one neurosurgeon in our group, but it makes no sense to send you to him when you're already in the care of another."

What made no sense was that all three of us were in Prairie Medical's office in Westwood, less than a mile from the UCLA clinic of Dr. Saxton—possibly the only specialist who could diagnose and treat me.

"But why can't you refer me to Dr. Filler—and Dr. Saxton, who he says can treat my crashes?" I desperately crammed her name into my question. Thomason was a decent man.

"I'm forbidden to refer you to anyone at UCLA," he answered gently.

"No one at the WGA told me," I said, as I tried to understand why no one at the Guild warned me of the true meaning of "UniversalCare."

"I expect the insurance brokers don't know,"

Thomason replied with finality, and waved us goodbye. "It was nice to meet you."

The business of caring that year stripped me of access to all UCLA doctors—Filler and Saxton alike—and even deprived me of access to my UCLA internist. As the next section of the path to recovery completely vanished, we called Lois for some emergency advice, and met for lunch next day. But although Lois was my guru for many things, she'd not heard of Dr. Saxton.

"How do I get into UCLA to see her, if Prairie is forbidden to send me there?" we asked over appetizers at a restaurant near her clinic. "Why doesn't Medicare work with a big hospital like UCLA?"

"They do," Lois countered, "just not that Prairie plan of yours."

As I was not to become his patient, Thomason proffered no explanation, no suggestion what I should do.

"So, Lois . . . there may be a way?" I couldn't see how. The WGA offered me no alternative to Prairie Medical.

"You have to get into a Medicare group at UCLA," Lois the guru said.

She sounded like Yoda in *Star Wars*, as he patiently explained rules of the cosmos to a confounded Luke Skywalker.

Join a UCLA Medicare group, you must, hmmm. . . .

And like Yoda, that's all Lois could say. Not how a person with disabilities could find one, or who to call. It took until the end of December to track down the right person.

"How do I get into a UCLA Medicare group?" I asked Tom, the Guild's insurance broker, careful to copy Lois's exact words. Like most everybody in the business of caring, once I found the right question and person to ask, he wanted to help.

"Call Health Net," he said.

"You've got to be kidding. Health Net just dropped me!"

"That's different," Tom replied. "Tell them you have Medicare, and you want an application packet for a UCLA group."

"But won't they reject me as soon as they see my claims history—*and* that they dropped me weeks ago?" Tom's suggestion sounded like a futile exercise.

"No, no," Tom chuckled. "Reps get paid very well for selling those policies."

"So . . . I ask for these forms, and I get to see my UCLA doctors?"

"Not quite," Tom said. I held my breath. "All you need is a primary care physician at UCLA, who's already in the group, to agree to take you."

That sounded easy enough. Tom's insight was the latest demonstration that no one tells you everything you need to know. I called Health Net's toll-free number, explained the urgency, and then followed Tom's instructions word for word. Just like he said, the carrier that had just dropped me readily sent the form. And also as Tom promised, on it there was a blank space for a primary care physician.

"Name of PCP?" it read. As the year ended, that empty space was all that separated me from all of UCLA's doctors, Dr. Saxton and my internist included. It turned out there were a very great number of doctors who either left UCLA, like Dr. Stone the shoulder specialist to get out of the system completely, or who remained in practice at the medical center, but refused to accept Medicare patients. I looked for all of 2003, and could not find a qualified specialist who'd put their name in that space. But at the start of 2004, my father, after many years with the brokerage firm Smith Barney, and my brother Jonathan—now one of their top

financial consultants—received great offers to move to
Wachovia Securities.

Under HIPAA—Clinton's health insurance portability law—my father had the right to transfer out of his
Smith Barney health plan to any of the groups offered
by his new employer. If he selected a UCLA group for
himself and my mother, there was a chance they could
include me as a family member, and bring me there too.
Our ever-helpful next-door neighbor, Harry the network
news producer, recommended a highly respected internist at UCLA. And on my father's acceptance into Wachovia's employee health plan, my parents requested an
urgent appointment, and drove over.

As soon as they signed in at Dr. Michael Brousseau's clinic with their own paperwork, they told his receptionist about me. They handed her my Health Net
form, complete and ready, save for Brousseau's signature
as my PCP in that solitary, long-empty blank space.

She looked it over, then handed it back.

"No, I'm afraid Dr. Brousseau isn't accepting any
Medicare patients," she explained quietly, like all the
others we tried.

My parents sat in the waiting room, heartbroken
and wondering how to tell me when they got home. A
few minutes later, Dr. Brousseau looked out his door at
his crestfallen new patients, and then came out.

"I don't split families," he said simply. "I'll take
Simon as well!"

It's not often your doctor saves your life before he
meets you, but that's how I felt when I met Dr. Brousseau for the initial consult. He was young, intelligent,
efficient, and above all, a doctor who had a heart. He
checked my files, reviewed my vital signs, and heard
about my desperate need to follow up Filler's long-
delayed recommendation to see Dr. Saxton about my
chronic headaches and crashes.

"You're still a complex case," he concluded. "I'll recommend you get a case manager to oversee that authorization."

"I had one before, Doctor, but she was in Colorado—"

"Ann Kingsley is a nurse here on campus," he interrupted, "with direct review of your files."

And when Ann reviewed them, she had UCLA authorize an initial consultation with Dr. Ernestina Saxton. There was no way to know if she might help, but with the long struggle won, I hoped I was headed in the right direction.

Like all good physicians, Dr. Saxton was incredibly busy, and it was early in February before my mother and I arrived at the large waiting room of UCLA's Department of Neurological Services. In due course, we graduated to the little room, which on first impression looked disappointingly identical to Filler's. Then I noticed something else: a computer monitor and keyboard. UCLA appeared to have moved its patient records online. That was something, I supposed, as the clock ticked on. After the long struggle to get into this room, somehow, without knowing quite what, I hoped for more. When she swept in to join us, Dr. Ernestina Saxton—or "you can call me Dolly!"—was a whole lot more. An intellectual firebrand of a doctor, she radiated expertise and dedication as she immediately pored over my records. She was appalled by Marcy's death, fascinated by my survival and recovery so far.

"My, my!" she exclaimed as I described the surgeries. She carefully reviewed the Arizona Dystonia Institute report, then Rancho's, and the others that described my symptoms.

"All these tests, you poor thing!" she clucked with genuine sympathy. "Let's have you keep a record of your crashes—start a migraine diary."

"But I don't have migraines," I objected, as I tried not to sound defensive.

"Patients never think they do!" Dolly answered with peals of laughter.

Her enthusiasm was contagious. If she could be so upbeat, maybe great things could happen in this small room with this ball of fire. I kept the migraine diary like she asked, the record of what I ate every meal before and what I did after I crashed. My crashes seemed random, and I worried that Dolly, my last hope, might give up on me. It looked headed that way at my follow-up.

"Nope, nothing here," she murmured absently as she leafed through pages of debilitating crashes and noted their frequency; I feared she was disappointed. Soon after she began her physical examination, a tall, powerfully built doctor slipped into our cubicle and sat on a chair, legs crossed, from where he watched us silently. What with the examination table, Dolly and her computer setup, my mother, myself, and our new addition with the physique of a football player, our cubicle felt as crowded as that Marx Brothers movie, when all the brothers stow away in the same ocean cabin. Except the tall stranger made no comment, and neither did Dolly. She continued her examination as if he wasn't there, lifted my arm into the air and with her other hand, cupped my chin, and then slowly turned my head.

"What do you feel?" she asked.

"I feel *okay*, but then I always feel like I'm not here," I added.

I did feel a little strange, it was true, but had for the last ten years. "You know, I totally crashed the day after Dr. Filler did something like this," I remembered aloud. My voice sounded a bit hollow, I thought. From low on the slope of consciousness surfaced a desire that I wanted to put my hand down, so I started to lower it.

"No," said Dolly, polite but firm. "How do you feel

now?"

How *did* I feel? How did *I* feel? *How* did I *feel*? I tried to think hard. So much depended on the answer.

"Um, I suppose the lighting in this room looks a little darker. . . ."

She released my arm. I was about to pass out, but with no awareness of that; the broken yardstick on display for all, except me, to see—my brain unable to measure itself. She began her other tests on my shoulders, spine, and pelvis until her recent arrival grew restless, and began to politely interrupt her.

"Yes, Dolly, scoliosis—with some atrophy!"

His forceful voice startled me. Though I heard him come in, he sat to my left in my blind spot where I couldn't see him, so silent I forgot he was there.

"This is Dr. James Collins," Dolly introduced the stranger.

"Hello, Lewis," he said gruffly.

It was hard to date him. Still wiry and energetic from his college athlete days, he explained how he was Dolly's professor when she started medical school at UCLA. His expertise was radiology, and as a full professor of it, he taught residents how to capture and read all kinds of diagnostic images. She explained my case history and family background, and Dr. Collins described with gusto, how his father's grandparents came from Ireland and Madagascar—"quite a combination!"—and how these forebears from such distant spots on the globe met at sea.

"I've a question, Lewis," he looked at me curiously. "What's two and two make?"

It might have seemed off track in a consult for migraine, but I figured he wanted to test my orientation.

"Four," I said thoughtfully.

"Sure of that?"

I thought a little more.

"I think so."

"Listen to yourself, and what you're saying," he eyed me mischievously. "What do you get if you add *two* and *two*?"

From the infinite matrix that is our minds, came a memory of a math teacher at King's College School in Wimbledon, and a story my brother David told me when he got home from school one day, thirty years before.

"Well," I puzzled, "if you're going to press me, then I'll say two and two can make *five*—for larger powers of two."

James Collins roared with a laugh that filled the room. The point was that if you always round numbers off, you miss the best answer. 2.4 + 2.4 comes to 4.8, to make a mathematical 5. But if you round each 2.4 *down* to 2, you would only ever get the result 4 and never see you have 5; you never see the full picture. I was relieved to solve the riddle, and move to the next level with Collins and Saxton.

"Here, Lewis," he held up an oversized envelope he'd brought to show his colleague, and drew out a long sheet of film. "Take a look at this MRA."

I'd never met a radiologist, only read their cryptic reports, and this one wanted to show me his latest work. My mother and I peered at a deep blood red view of a patient's torso that reminded me of Edvard Munch's *The Scream*, his picture of a man with hands raised to his head, eyes staring, mouth agape. This MRA of a young woman looked like a frozen scream, capturing an incredible still life of the inner structure, the inner beauty, of her whole upper body; the agony and ecstasy of one moment of her life.

"In every MRI, you've had," Dr. Collins continued, "the techs told you to lie still because movement ruins the picture, right?"

I nodded, remembered many such instructions, in so many inconclusive MRIs.

"Well years ago, I wondered if there was a way to harness that. Tune the MRI to measure the movement!"

My blank look must have shown I hadn't picked up what he put down. Collins went into teaching mode, like I was one of his medical school students.

"Tune it to the blood flow! I started to put a saline water bag in the tunnel alongside the patient years ago, to tune the machine to all those concentrated hydrogen protons!"

Maybe he saw the question in my eyes.

"Why's it matter so much? I'll tell you something medical school teaches every resident in first year anatomy: your body *has one circulation system. . . ."*

I remembered Dr. Zhong and her assistant Beth and how they talked about *qi*, the one circulation of Chinese medicine.

"And then, doctors break our circulation into separate components and specialize," he said with regret. "Pulmonary circulation . . . coronary . . . systemic—and forget what they first learned." I tried to keep up.

"I was told a compressed nerve is like a squashed garden hose, and I need to release it. That's why Dr. Filler—"

"Nerves and blood together. That's the one system," Dr. Collins interrupted. "Blood flows around in your body, and your nerves are wrapped around it."

He was the first Western doctor I met to link my nerves and blood together.

"So, Lewis," he accelerated to his conclusion, "if there's compression at one point in the blood's circulation—someone's stepped on the garden hose as you put it—it has to expand someplace else in your body's sealed system. And wherever it does, it presses on those surrounding nerves and causes pain. To ease your pain, you must find where your blood flow is compressed."

His logic was compelling.

"I expect you're very tired, and have to go to bed in the morning after you shower?" he offered with a smile.

Dr. Collins was also the first Western doctor to describe a symptom before I did. "Keep your hands below your head when you wash your hair—and when you dry it."

He already had my trust, but I couldn't see how the two were connected or had anything to do with my crashes and a squashed hosepipe.

"Um, okay, but why will that help?" I asked cautiously.

"See here," Collins pointed again to the torso on the young woman's MRA. I saw a faint outline.

"You mean that?"

"No, that's her liver!" he snapped impatiently. *"That . . ."*

He tapped his powerful fingers on what looked so insignificant amongst the glorious beauty of that human form, it didn't seem possible they meant anything at all: some tiny white marks in her abdomen.

"You mean those specks?" I asked nervously. I didn't want to antagonize this doctor Dolly admired, and who might put me back on the hidden path.

"Yes, those specks," he playfully mimicked, as though nothing could be more obvious.

"This patient suffers terrible migraine headaches, and those specks show *where* her blood flow's compressed. She feels her pain *not* at the compression point way down there by her liver," Collins continued, as his hand began to trace upwards, "but where that pressure makes the vessels bulge in response—and press on the surrounding nerves higher up *in her head.*"

His hand came to a rest directly over the skull of

this young woman in constant pain.

"Release that pressure—and no more migraine!"

I remembered all the vague words in my neurologists' reports: "*consistent* with . . ." and "*possible*," the nonspecific language doctors use so no patient can pin them down to a definite diagnosis.

"Sure," Collins agreed, "we've had patients with a dozen surgeries on their nerves who are still in pain because no one identified where the compression was."

Dr. Collins had the compression map in his hand and just shown me, a layman, the critical junctions, the points in a hundred thousand miles of blood vessels that were the definitive cause of a symptom. With it, he'd illuminated the key this woman sought in the darkness within her. I was filled with the most wonderful sensation for those who seek the path to full recovery. It was certainty that I was in the right place, with two great doctors who could evaluate me, head to tail, in the search for my key.

"Dr. Collins," Dolly asked, "isn't your patient waiting?"

He waved his hand impatiently with the passion of a research scientist. "It's okay—she's in anesthesia."

Dr. Saxton's question made me desperately aware how short time was.

"If the car crash squashed my blood vessels, so pressure on the hose pipes makes them bulge someplace else in my body," I struggled, as I frantically tried to make his solution connect with my problems, "I'd have high blood pressure, wouldn't I?"

I suddenly wished I thought my question through before I began. Surely my next words would end this man's interest, rule me out for treatment when I so badly wanted him to take one of those torso pictures, and make a map for me. My shoulders sagged as I confessed.

"But I don't have high blood pressure, Doctor. In

fact it's very *low*, so I can't have compression like the woman in your picture." I looked up sadly at Collins and Saxton, who didn't look that way at all.

"Which means," Collins said with growing excitement, "that it's very low *where they take it!*"

"They take it on my arm," I observed, a statement of the obvious, while I tried to figure out what he meant.

"So," he explained patiently, "all those readings tell you that your blood pressure is very low *in your arm.*"

First inklings of comprehension trickled in.

"And," Dr. Collins pressed, "you really, really hate it when they take your blood pressure, don't you? Can't wait for them to take the cuff off your arm, am I right?"

I looked at him in disbelief and wondered how he could possibly know that too, any more than how I went back to bed every morning after my shower.

"It's hard for you because your blood flow's already compromised, and the cuff restricts it even worse," he explained nonchalantly. "The point, Lewis, is this: If we could take your blood pressure *exactly where your garden hose is compressed?*" he looked at me inquiringly, a test of whether his student kept up.

"It would be . . . high?" I managed.

"Through the roof!" he exclaimed enthusiastically, and beamed at me. "I'll see you in radiology!" Then he vanished to attend to his patient.

My mother and I exchanged looks with Dolly at his magic final words. The man who understood how two and two make five would image my blood flow. All my attention was on it until I arrived for what would, in Dr. Collins's hands, be an MRI, MRA, and MRV.

I listened to the cloppety-clop sound of horses' hooves patter past my head in the tunnel for an eternity, a saline water bag at my side, and wondered how deep into the mysteries of my body, the mysteries of life, this remarkable man could reach. I wondered more when I heard his gravelly voice on the intercom.

"Lewis, hands over your head!" the pallet slid out, and Collins initiated a completely fresh imaging series in the tunnel.

"Any symptoms in that position?" he quizzed some time later.

I couldn't feel a difference, any more than when I started to pass out in Dolly's office.

"That's okay!" James's voice rang cheerfully through the tunnel, his study complete. "Come in here when you're changed."

No radiologist shared their images with me before, let alone invited me to their console after an examination. My mother and I sat with Dr. Collins as massive computers compiled the unimaginable quantities of data necessary to yield the positions of all those individual atoms, at a level of accuracy to give him his calculated "Fives."

"Why do invertebrates *not* sleep?" James asked the room while the hard drives and fans whirred.

As an animal that often slept twelve hours straight, then some more after his morning shower, I couldn't imagine any animal that didn't sleep at all.

"To not get eaten," he answered his own question, and turned to me.

"So, why *do* vertebrates like us sleep?"

I thought I should be able to answer that one.

"Because . . . I know I *won't* get eaten?" I tried.

"No, Lewis!"

He shook his head at my ignorance.

"No, you sleep to dream and—by dreaming—to learn from the day."

It was, I realized, something I did ever since the accident, even in my coma.

"That's how I became interested in radiology in

the first place," he continued, "to search for the totality of life and learn from it."

It reminded me after so many years why I first came to filmmaking, which, like our dreams, seeks to weave something interesting and helpful from the daily rush of life.

Dr. Collins observed that things happen for a reason, and I said I couldn't accept that, because it's unfair to those who lose by it: the injured, the sick, and the dead.

"There's an ancient story I want you to think about," James said, "of a man in a Jamaican village who travels a safe path through the jungle every day. The voodoo witch doctor warns him, 'You'll meet a skeleton on that path and die!'"

He expertly downloaded more images to process.

"So, one day as the man walks along his path, he thinks he sees the skeleton in the distance coming toward him. He remembers the witch doctor's warning, so he leaves his usual path to avoid it, and off his usual path, falls into quicksand and dies!"

His point made, Dr. Collins focused all his attention on the console.

I thought I understood. Whether the way through the jungle was the path of life that ends in death, or the hidden one to full recovery, there are many choices to make along it that we must confront. Stay on the path at all costs, and face whatever we meet on it, no matter the consequences. And James already saw my next choices in the skeleton images he compiled on his monitors.

By good fortune, he and Dolly were to fly to a medical conference in Florida the next morning. Having decided to present my case there, he needed to rehearse his presentation right then. My father knew my mother and I arrived at 4:00 PM, so when he entered the radiology clinic at 7:00 PM he expected, quite reasonably, to find

us ready to leave. Instead, Dr. Collins was just about
to start. He could not have asked for a more attentive
audience. He explained how he derived these images;
how every choice, from which slices to take to the exact
degree of spin on the protons to which particular magnetic coils to harness, shapes the images that emerge.
I imagined Dr. Collins as a conductor who knew how
to tune a vast electronic orchestra to attain a perfect
note, and now prepared to show us his masterpiece: a
vivid demonstration of the guesswork of neurosurgery
by other doctors, and the cutting edge possibilities of diagnosis with the "five" data of his MRA that I glimpsed
in Dolly's clinic.

His presentation to the audience the next day followed, of data overlooked by doctors and surgeons alike
for over ten years.

"This is a simple diagnosis," he began, "of a forty-
six-year-old male. . . ."

A simple diagnosis. . . .

My parents and I were rapt as a screen showed
the exact data slices Dr. Collins imaged; from where on
each side of my torso he obtained these two-dimensional, high-resolution MRI cuts in four planes that revealed
my blood vessels in high resolution, as a delicate white
latticework.

"There are the primary blood vessels," he intoned,
as massive computer drives processed data, "and here,
the secondaries. In two-dimensional analysis, it appears
that on both your left and right sides, you have signifi-
cantly reduced blood supply in the primary system, and
the engorged secondaries suggest those vessels have attempted to substitute—unsuccessfully."

He turned to us.

"So we think you have bilateral thoracic outlet
syndrome, Simon. Your first rib on both sides presses
on your carotid and jugular—and cuts the blood supply

to your head."

"Is that why I felt so good for a while after hyperbaric oxygen—more oxygen could get through?" I asked.

"Of course, of course. . . ." Dr. Collins quickly prepared his data to prove this initial two-dimensional assessment to tomorrow's audience, and as the main show began, and software interpolation allowed him to create a three-dimensional image reconstruction, a walk through the nerve-blood system of this forty-six-year-old male began to emerge. I saw how blood vessels gracefully curved their way past organs and muscles, brought oxygen, and took away carbonic acid. He showed my blood vessels as they arrived, full, on *one* side of the bicuspid valve by my broken ribs and collarbone, but emerged depleted on the other.

"Proving compression *right there. . . .*"

Dr. Collins switched to images in my shoulder, where blood vessels pressed against their surrounding nerves, far removed from my fingers and hands, numb and tingling ever since the crash.

"*And there.*" The combined two- and three-dimensional images proved his diagnosis, and were a total review of my condition. I had double thoracic outlet syndrome—compression in the life-critical space where blood and nerves enter and leave the head. It was 8:00 PM when we left, exhausted but rejuvenated and excited. I found Collins only through Dr. Filler's referral to Dr. Saxton, so perhaps Filler was my deus ex machina after all.

In August, I saw Dr. Saxton to discuss my treatment, and James came in soon after we began. For thoracic outlet surgery, they explained, a highly specialized test was required first, called a scalene block, and "a doctor called Endiman" was one of the very few who performed it.

"Do you know him?" Dolly inquired.

I felt I'd worked my way through almost everyone in town—or more to the point, they'd worked their
way through me.

"Saw him for the piriformis surgeries!" I replied.
If I'd met all the top nerve specialists in L.A., I reflected,
it looked as if this might be the final team of my recovery with, it appeared, one final player.

"If Endiman's nerve block confirms," Dr. Saxton
said, "we'll refer you to Sam Ahn."

Off my inquiring look she added, "He's a vascular
surgeon—to evaluate resection of your first rib."

However much it might help, it was still hard to
hear I needed to lose a rib.

"To give your neurovascular bundle more room,"
Dolly added as encouragement. I comforted myself that
Dr. Ahn would be my last surgeon, as I left with the
detailed MRA report Collins gave me. Regardless of the
ultimate outcome, I knew I was on the hidden path once
more. As I contemplated the removal of ribs required
for my next step along it, the phone rang one afternoon.
It was Marcy's closest friend.

"Hi Simon!" Tova shouted through the wind noise
of her cell, as if it was ten days since we last spoke, instead of ten years.

"Where are you, Tova?" I asked in wonder.

"About five minutes from your house!"

Minutes later, I limped out to meet Tova in her
white Mazda Miata convertible as it pulled in front, almost a match for my RX-7 still parked in my parents'
garage. Tova's golden retriever Maggie was at her side
for her journey from her family in Phoenix to her home
in San Francisco. On impulse, Tova detoured south
through L.A. to see how I was.

Reassurance that my old life still existed couldn't
have come at a better time, as we talked about past and

future, and Tova gave me her cell number. We hugged, Tova's tires squealed from the curb and I waved good-bye as she sped down our street, Maggie's ears flapping in the wind.

Tova's life of easy mobility and choice reminded me of my isolation, and the unlimited promise of the freedom that comes with full recovery, but later that month I suffered a crash that lasted two weeks. That alone wasn't too much of a surprise, but by the end of it my eyes couldn't open, which was a big, bad one.

"Edema—we don't like fluid near the eyes," Dr. Brousseau said tersely, and ordered emergency CT scans of my sinuses. An immediate consultation followed with a youthful, bright, and personable UCLA specialist, who looked briefly at the scans then carefully read the report. He seemed to be very competent, very *together*. Based on the report, Doctor Together said there were two possible surgeries, but suggested I try nasal spray first. I asked to see the report Doctor Together relied on.

"The frontal sinuses are opacified," the radiologist began. And concluded that "the remainder of the examination is *unremarkable*." It was the same word the unobservant radiologist used of my absent gallbladder. I made a mental note to ask Dr. Saxton for her opinion, after I met Dr. Ahn.

At the end of September, my mother and I waited in reception to see him at UCLA's Gonda Vascular Center. It's a hard time for a patient; you hope the surgeon can help, but worry what will happen next if they can. So I sat and wondered what a vascular surgeon could do for something called thoracic outlet syndrome, when Dr. James Collins happened by.

"Lewis! Mrs. Lewis! Who are you here to see?"

As we told him, Dr. Collins described more about his research, and about the millions of dollars that this great university funded to make his special scans possible.

"Now, don't forget, Lewis—shake your hands," James reminded me, as he gestured goodbye.

I looked back at him blankly.

"To restore circulation when you need it."

I'd forgotten his simple, useful tip.

"And tell Sam to lighten up!" he laughed, as he went on his way.

Minutes later, I understood. Dr. Sam Ahn, extremely quiet and disconcertingly serious, was a vascular surgeon who specialized in rib resections. By this point, I was used to doctors who wanted to raise my arm and turn my head, and dreaded the crash I would suffer that night and next day. He seemed noncommittal about what he could hear through his stethoscope as he raised each arm and listened. I didn't care; Collins walked me through my body on his screens—I'd seen *inside*. I was also ready for the mantra.

"Can you live with this—the way you are?" Dr. Ahn began.

I hadn't expected this new version. Because of the damage to my mind, I was none too sure how I felt from one moment to the next. To answer his question, I tried to imagine what life would be like without crashes, and realized that, after ten years of disability and surgery, I couldn't remember how a normal healthy one felt any more. I thought of my brother Jonathan's new baby boy Sammy, of hopes for the future.

"If I was eighty-five," I finally said, "*yes*, I could accept how I am. But I'm forty-six, and *no*, I can't go on like this."

"It's a very serious surgery, to take out a rib. You might die," he pointed out grimly.

I was back on familiar terrain.

"I understand, Doctor—could you do both?"

It wasn't bravery, or bravado; it was easier to face death once rather than twice. And I knew Dr. Johnson had flipped me to remove bone from both sides of my pelvis.

"No way," Dr. Ahn replied. "We can only resect one rib at a time. Which side would you like first?"

I weighed which shoulder and arm mattered most.

"Take the right rib first," I answered. It would be the worst side to lose if something went wrong, but I picked it because my body was most likely better developed on that side, with more room for him to work and a better chance of success. Although I knew Dr. Ahn was my next step on the path, I began to panic by the time I saw Dolly at my next consult.

"And how was Dr. Ahn?" asked Dr. Saxton brightly.

"Well, he was so *somber.* . . ."

"And what did you say?"

"That it's one thing if you're eighty-five and another if you're forty-six."

"Good for you!" she agreed enthusiastically. "You want the relief. . . ."

Her comment brought me back into the simplest focus, and my questions.

"I asked him to take my right rib first, Doctor. Was that okay?"

"Well," Dolly burst into an encouraging laugh, "we always say deal with your worst problem first, so if you get hit by a truck after, at least you got the most benefit while you could!" Perhaps she saw me flinch. "Oh!" she corrected herself quickly, and smiled, "I can't believe I said that—I forgot you already were hit by a truck!"

Dolly was the greatest. And she was about to prove it again, because my next question was to follow up my note to ask her about my "unremarkable" sinus study. After all, the sinuses were in my head, and like Dr. Collins said, there was only one circulation system in us. In contrast with Doctor Together, who focused most of his attention on the radiologist's typed report, I saw Dolly, as I began my question, turn away to her computer screen, pull reports off it, review all the work over the years at UCLA, and then very carefully inspect the new CT scan images for herself. Just like Dr. Collins and Dr. Filler, she wanted to decide for herself, with her own eyes, whether or not the study was *unremarkable*.

"Opacity . . . that's how bad you are," she murmured.

I got to the end of my story, and Doctor Together's suggestion of nose spray as first choice. She was unequivocal.

"You don't want to use a spray. This could be the cause of a lot of your pain," was her very different diagnosis.

Dr. Saxton still gazed at the CT images on her light panel that revealed so much to her, hummed quietly to herself and then turned back to us.

"Daniel Castro," she said simply, "he's the man to see."

Without further ado, she dialed his office on her speakerphone to set the earliest possible appointment, as my mother and I watched in awe.

"This is Portia," announced the bright and strong voice of Dr. Castro's office coordinator, who found she was trapped out in the open on a speakerphone between doctor and patient, the normally hidden barriers of the business of caring exposed.

"We . . . uh, we . . . can't see HMO patients here," she said awkwardly, and our hopes collapsed as we once again confronted the Byzantine rules of modern healthcare. My family's hard-won insurance that got me in via

Dr. Brousseau to see Dr. Saxton at UCLA in the first place, for some reason, wasn't enough to see the next UCLA specialist I needed. Once more, the business of caring seemed to change the rules and block access.

"But I'm a complex case; I have a case manager— Ann Kingsley," I pleaded, a sudden groping thought that sprang from desperation. "Can't my case manager get authorization?"

There was silence on the speaker line, as the co-ordinator checked the name.

"Ah, here's Ann Kingsley at UCLA," came her voice at last. "With a case manager . . . and Medicare . . . we *can* get you in!"

I could scarcely believe her instant one-eighty as my path reopened. Not only did Dr. Saxton's level of investigation turn a four into five, but I'd also found a doctor who might cure the violent crashes in my head. It was another moment of transition, from darkness into the light, except now there were two surgeons lined up.

"Um, what about Sam Ahn?" I already had an appointment with Dr. Endiman in two weeks, to do the special diagnostic test Dr. Ahn required before he could take out my rib, and any delay might push it into the insurance uncertainty of the new year.

"Who goes first?" I added.

I forgot Dr. Castro's coordinator was still on the line.

"When's the nerve block with Endiman?" her voice asked through the speaker.

"October twenty-eighth."

"Dr. Castro will see you on the twenty-fifth. Just make sure you get Ann's paperwork to us," Portia said, in a different tone. For now, it was the voice of welcome.

CHAPTER NINETEEN

AN OPEN MIND

What lies behind us and what lies before us are tiny matters compared to what lies within us.

—Ralph Waldo Emerson

Three days before Dr. Endiman's nerve block, it was a record-breaking wait for my first consultation at Dr. Daniel Castro's clinic. Our appointment was at noon, and now it was after 4:00 PM. From time to time, someone, presumably Dr. Castro, hammered once on a cubicle door, his signal to the duty nurse he was done with that patient. Occasionally, his distant voice murmured instructions. A nurse deposited some examination instruments on a tray in our room, and then even the thumps stopped.

Time spent waiting for answers doesn't matter so long as you get them, and I had a lot of hopes pinned on Dr. Castro, whose card showed he was a professor of "nasal/sinus sleep disorders, oncology and lasers."

"Helloooo, Mister . . . Lewis, is it?" came a lilting accent from the door, and jolted me awake. A kindly gray-haired man smiled at me from the threshold to the cubicle.

"So sorry for the wait."

He promptly left, for so long I began to wonder if I imagined his momentary appearance. When Dr. Castro finally returned, he studied all my scans intently, followed by examination with a light at the tip of a very long probe that reminded me of E.T. in the movie, when he held up his long lighted finger—especially when my eyes saw an image of a red glowing orb. Who'd have guessed E.T. the extra-terrestrial was an intergalactic sinus expert, come to cure us all.

Compared with Doctor Together, it was a different level of examination, and Dr. Castro never mentioned nose spray.

"We need to open the doors," he sighed gently.

"The doors?" I asked involuntarily.

It struck me how many I had to open to find the hidden path to my recovery, and was curious what he meant.

"Our sinuses are eight doors into the brain. We must open some."

How many was "some," I wondered, but was too grateful for his diagnosis and solution to ask. Portia booked Dr. Castro's surgery right after Dr. Endiman's test, for which I arrived three days later. As he inserted an IV, Endiman explained how the nerve block was a dress rehearsal for rib removal—a glimpse of how I'd be after. His probe inserted deep, I heard the dry crackling of nerves within my body, as he asked me to open and close my fingers. They felt warmer, my arm less numb.

"You'll benefit from rib resection," he nodded, "so I'll recommend it to Ahn."

It was hard not to feel disappointed, not to wonder if it happened at all, when the good sensations disappeared in the time it took to leave his clinic and reach my mother's car. When I read the nerve block report, which was filled with caution and ambiguity, I remembered the one Collins gave me, the diagnostic certainty that showed the way forward.

The evening before Dr. Castro would "open some of the doors," the phone rang. It was Doctor Feelgood, who conscientiously called to discuss my drugs for next morning. After I checked into UCLA Medical Center, he showed up beside my gurney with his weight-watcher's question, but having carefully listened to my past difficulties the night before, elected to use a special IV needle.

"*This one!*" he announced with pride, a marksman with his weapon of choice. The last time I saw a needle that big was on a nature documentary, when the gamekeeper loaded a tranquilizer dart for a rhino, but it meant the massive device went in on his first attempt. It was time for Feelgood to drop his drug, and make me feel *goood*. The worst was over.

A woman approached, in a multicolored clown's bib, and it struck me this was another surgery on Halloween.

"Mr. Lewis," she announced in a ghostly whisper, "you have to *take this*."

She revealed a small medical vial, and then continued as if telling a ghost story.

"It's really, really *disgusting*," she shared, "but you know who's to blame? Dr. Castro!"

I wondered how disgusting it could possibly be— after all, I even came to like the taste of Dr. Zhong's incredibly bitter Chinese herbal tea—then realized something very curious. She said I had to take the vial . . . not drink it.

Dread of the immediate unknown loomed toward me out of Feelgood's purple haze. I yearned for him to press his oversized plunger. *Take me away and bring me back.*

The vial was disgusting as promised, as my cheerful visitor poured the ugly liquid into my nose, to who knew where.

"Thanks for warning me," I mumbled. "Nurses usually sugarcoat it."

My Halloween clown took it well. "Maybe that's because I'm not your nurse!" she laughed. "I'm Dr. Koster."

I smiled back wanly. "Um, well thanks, Doctor, all the same. . . ."

And having prepped me, she left. When she returned, the ward anesthesiologist wasn't smiling.

"I can't approve you for surgery, Mr. Lewis. There's a problem with your heart," Dr. Koster said with finality, and began to shut down the IV.

I couldn't accept my cancelation, not after I endured Feelgood's gargantuan IV, and her disgusting vial down my nose. I'd *earned my passage* on this trip. Packed my bags and was ready for takeoff.

"I have benign—" I attempted.

"There's no such thing as benign sick sinus syndrome," she interrupted, "but if Bersohn's positive report is in the system we can pull it."

I lay and waited as she disappeared to search UCLA's database; envied the other patients already on their happy trips in nearby operating rooms. Whatever came next, I didn't want to go home with the doors in my head still closed.

Dr. Koster reappeared with a bleak expression. "Report's not in the system," she said pensively.

"I'm sure I'll be okay, Doctor," I coaxed, and tried to sound more confident than I felt.

"Hmm," she checked my chart. "Well, you survived a whole day of surgery with Dr. Filler. . . ."

"And I'm sure I'll survive this too, Doctor," I begged, as my eyes urged her on. She almost shrugged, gave me yet another patient consent form to sign to protect the hospital if I died, and cleared me for takeoff. Dr. Castro came by, gowned for surgery and curious where his patient had gotten to.

"Which side is worse, Simon?" he inquired softly.

I'd thought a lot about the eight doors he showed me into my brain, into my consciousness. "Er, my left side, but, Doctor?"

"Yeeees?" that kind, lilting voice again.

"Every surgery—it's always turned out worse than they thought . . . ," I began.

He looked at me intently over his mask.

"So, please," I said, "whatever the risk . . . open as many doors as you can."

To treat this legacy of my head injury, undiagnosed in my sinuses for ten years, Dr. Castro performed six surgical procedures, followed after discharge by an almost overwhelming course of multiple drugs and irrigation. It was as if a dam had opened behind my forehead. By night, I slept fitfully with powerful dreams in blazing color that switched on and off, psychedelic designs and memories in complete detail from as far back as my college rooms at Cambridge.

It was in this heightened state that I accepted an invitation from David Irving, brother of actress Amy Irving and director of a movie I produced. David was chair of undergraduate film at the Tisch School of the Arts in New York, and invited me to a fundraising gala attended by major stars and other leaders in the creative community. David wanted to help me re-enter the flow of the film business, but I felt euphoric and disoriented at the table. As I tried to appear lucid, I wondered if the open doors in my head showed in my eyes; what my dinner partners thought of me and my role in their world after ten disabled years.

Medicare had the same question, and later that month, my mother brought me to the local Social Security office for my next Continuing Disability Review. As Medicare was my only health insurance, my recovery depended on their decision.

The interview was conducted by a man who was disabled himself. The question asked without words was why, if this case manager came to work every day in spite of his challenges, I couldn't. My interviewer, a quiet man in his late fifties, was in a wheelchair. They lost my file, he explained, and asked me to fill in a fresh form, instead of the one I completed at home with my parents' help.

With great difficulty, he pushed the blank form toward me across his desk. My eyes and face still swam from Dr. Castro's surgery. As I tried to focus, my interviewer asked how I earned the income declared on one of my tax returns since the crash.

"How much . . . income . . . was there?" I asked, tremulous in the suddenly oppressive silence of the government office.

"Let's see, Mr. Lewis. . . ."

He adjusted the endless papers before him awkwardly with one hand, and eventually looked up.

"Seventy-two cents."

It baffled me. But then I remembered a bar in L.A. where actors pin their residual checks for less than a dollar on the wall. The seventy-two cents, I told him, must be a residual check for acting in my first film, where I played a cameo role. It was stifling in the office, and my interviewer closed his eyes as a small fan tried to move the air. Perhaps his disabilities made it hard for him to keep awake—it was often impossible for me—or maybe he watched me still. I struggled, and couldn't co-ordinate my hands and eyes, or cope with the information the form asked; so many surgeries, so much pain.

We'd waited a long time for the interview, the form was very long, and eventually, I asked to go to the bathroom. My interviewer pointed, gave directions to it three times, and then understood I couldn't follow them.

"Perhaps it would be better if you went with Simon," he said to my mother.

When the letter came with Social Security's decision, it said I was permanently disabled, subject to review in another three years.

At my follow-up, it was clear that, like most busy surgeons, Dr. Castro was ready to move on. I thought his focus might shift today, so I was prepared for my three minutes with him. I knew I couldn't withstand another head surgery after this latest, and was determined to make this man tell me how to anticipate relapses, and avoid them.

"I didn't know I had all this infection before, Dr. Castro. How will I know in future if the problem is back?" That was a good question, I thought.

"Ah, we go with the symptoms," was his soft evasion. But one of his rehab instructions was to sleep at night half-reclined on several pillows temporarily. I tried that route.

"What about sleeping position long term?"

"Ummm, must elevate the bed."

My mother and I quickly coaxed the information that I should raise the head of my bed; that only four inches might suffice, and I could use two 2 × 4s nailed together like a brick, so the bed remained stable. Castro seemed to lean toward the door, as if there was a force field about to suck him from the cubicle; my time was up. The heck with social niceties, I waited hours for this.

"Is there anything else I should do? *Long term?*"

"Ah, the ocean . . . ," he mumbled indistinctly.

He was on his way out of the room—until my mother intercepted him for details. The "Ocean" in question was an over-the-counter product, a simple saline solution. I followed all of Dr. Castro's suggestions. My father nailed the wood together on the garage floor, and the saline spray was as pleasant as a walk on the beach to breathe the salt air. I was shortly to learn the level of Castro's skill from Dr. Saxton.

"This . . . is . . . *huge*," she breathed, as she read every line of the multipage operation report, reciting each sinus, each door into my mind, that Dr. Castro opened—for he took me at my word, and opened all eight. "We need to see if we can fix you, like the bionic man. Put you back together—one piece at time!"

"Well, I saw Dr. Endiman for his test, and he said I've got thoracic outlet syndrome."

"Good," Dolly said.

She picked up her phone to set my next appointment right then, with Sam Ahn.

"I've a question, Dolly," I blurted. I might not see her again before Ahn's surgery, and wondered how I might get the best experience with Doctor Feelgood.

"Garbage," she answered, simply. "Ask for the garbage."

Every anesthetic in Feelgood's arsenal gave side effects so, Dolly continued, if you mixed them up you got a "garbage anesthetic," a cocktail that diluted them.

"A little of every side effect, instead of a whole lot of one of them," she finished.

The depression tidal wave I felt after some surgeries was one side effect, throwing up in the recovery room another. After so many surgeries, I knew something productive I could ask Doctor Feelgood, and felt more confident until I saw Dr. Ahn, who was now authorized to discuss surgical resection of my right rib.

I understood why Collins warned me, as Dr. Ahn explained this might not help my hands, how they might be paralyzed, that the whole enterprise was "real risky," and I might die. He drew a diagram of where he'd cut into me at the top of my ribcage; how, if he nicked *this* nerve, my arm would be paralyzed for the rest of my life, or *this* nerve, and I'd never again take a normal breath.

"How much do you want to take those risks?" he asked.

Because of my visual deficits, I couldn't understand Dr. Ahn's anatomically correct drawing, or link it with my body, so had no clue where he would go in, or how my rib would come out.

"I understand, Doctor," I said. "Let's do it."

Bersohn, my cardiologist, had me wear another twenty-four-hour Holter to check my heart for the operation, while my internist Dr. Brousseau also wanted me to understand the extent of the risk.

"I have a patient who was left with an arm like a chicken wing, it stuck out sideways," he warned. "She couldn't lower it to her side!"

That horrified, but didn't deter, me. I asked Dr. Brousseau to run a full EKG as well as the Holter to avoid another heart-related delay with Feelgood. And then, my preparations complete, I counted the days.

Because I asked to be Dr. Ahn's first surgery, I had a 4:30 AM report time. It's difficult to prepare to have a functional part of you taken away, so I stared blankly through the window as my mother drove, increasingly disassociated from the world around me as we pulled into Santa Monica-UCLA Medical Center, completed paperwork, and checked into a shared room for insertion of my IV. The nurse arrived to take my roommate first, and I envied him a little because he'd go under before me.

"And what are you here for today?" the cheerful

nurse's voice rang through a superfluous privacy curtain.

"Operation on my left testicle," his strained reply, accompanied by way more information about it than I needed to know just then. Suddenly I didn't feel envious, more like shamefully grateful I was only to lose a rib. The very experienced IV nurse plugged me in smooth and easy, and my mother stayed to keep me safe. By this point, we both knew the need for constant vigilance, and she wouldn't leave my side even for the few minutes that remained until transportation took me down to surgery.

5:30 AM passed silently. My testicular neighbor was long gone. I'd become invisible like Mr. Cellophane in the musical *Chicago*. Nurses walked right by our door, looked right past us, and couldn't see us.

"We can't operate on Simon today," the floor nurse explained, after my mother searched her out on the ward, and practically dragged her into my room.

"There's a question about his heart."

I was too stressed to speak.

"This always comes up," my mother took over for me evenly. "He just had major sinus surgery in October, and Dr. Koster specially cleared him for that."

I remembered Halloween bib's casual shrug. All I needed was one of those.

"No," the nurse insisted. "We can't proceed with the ribectomy."

"You must! We've brought Dr. Brousseau's EKG, *and* his report, *and* the complete printout from Bersohn's twenty-four-hour Holter!" my mother's voice rose, desperate and shrill in the quiet hospital, "What more about his heart could you possibly want?"

The nurse wilted, but stood her ground.

"We don't have Dr. Bersohn's specific report that approves Mr. Lewis for *this* surgery," she explained, then finally acknowledged there was a patient in the room, and turned her attention to Mr. Cellophane.

"We have to send you home, Mr. Lewis," she concluded.

Once again trapped by the fact that no one tells you everything, even when you think you've asked the right questions, I started to break down.

"If I leave, I'm not coming back," I sobbed. It was a childish threat. If my heart was too weak, they'd not let me back, and no one else would take me either.

"You wait right there!" my mother ordered the nurse, as she dialed my father. He'd relied on Dr. Bersohn for years and knew the right emergency number. At 6:30 AM, Bersohn sent a hard copy of his opinion of my heart condition to our floor nurse, who waited by the fax.

"The whole team's standing by," a transportation intern explained as he instantly wheeled me into the hall, spun my gurney toward the OR, and paused, to let the patient exchange last thoughts with his family.

"Goodbye, Mom," was all I could muster, with a hug. On my long drive to the hospital to give up a rib and risk death, the only way I found to cope was in acceptance that today was the day I might die. It was easier to say goodbye in the hall, relinquish my life here, to pick up again with infinite gratitude if and when I woke.

"Oh, no," the goodhearted intern broke in. "How about, 'I'll see you later'?"

He popped a paper hat with an elastic band on my head, like I was headed to a child's birthday party, and whisked me top speed through the patient-only doors. Showtime for Doctor Feelgood also, who appeared at my side.

"A hundred and seventy pounds," I cut across his question. "And Dr. Saxton said to ask you for the garbage anesthetic," I added hurriedly.

In mid-step, Feelgood gave a big smile and promptly dropped his usual speech.

"Oh, *yes!*" he said with the evident pleasure of a chef when conversation turns to recipes with a knowledgeable customer. "Everything here comes straight out of the garbage pail!"

Accepting that I might die made these last crumbs of interaction precious.

"And I'd like please to not throw up in the recovery room."

"Okay," he said amiably. This culinary master was up to special orders. "I'll leave out the opioid. You'll be more lucid in the OR, but shouldn't throw up after."

"Thanks, Doctor, that will be great."

After one of the worst starts, this was the best Feelgood conversation yet. I noticed the hall was only five feet high now, the roof curved, like a tunnel. This was some *goood* garbage.

"Ahh, so glad you could make it!" a masked and gowned Dr. Ahn welcomed me with his team in the operating room, complete with bright overhead lights. As Feelgood promised, I was still lucid, and when Dr. Ahn leaned over me, I saw he wore goggles.

"Put a pair on him," he instructed, and a team member fitted me with the tightest pair I ever wore outside of a swimming pool. In my paper hat and goggles, I felt quite at home; now I looked like one of the team.

Feelgood applied a mask, and I breathed pure oxygen. Comforting memories flowed of the hyperbaric chamber, and from my coma on life support beyond. I no longer felt stress, as Feelgood started to take it—and me—away. I noticed Dr. Ahn tug my right arm.

"Tell me, Mr. Lewis," he asked innocently, "if I pull your arm like this, does it dislocate?"

"Um, no, I don't think so," I replied as I looked up at Sam.

I looked down again in time to watch my right arm move away from me to a strange place.

"Hmm . . . sssneakyyy," I mumbled. I heard the team's laughter, and drifted gently away.

Consciousness returned slowly in the recovery room, aware only that I was alive, and not that I still had a Jackson-Pratt inside me, to drain blood from my deep surgical wound. I felt one nausea wave, didn't throw up, and was more than grateful. I felt sensations of an adrenaline rush mingled with depression. Just like Dolly promised, you got a diluted version of everything from a garbage anesthetic.

"Hi, Simon!"

I looked up to the beautiful eyes of a very familiar face. It was great to see her, though I was too weak to place her name.

"Connie," she prompted, smiling. "I saw your name on the list and had to see if it was really you!"

Never was an old friend a more welcome sight than my nurse from the hyperbaric chamber, who decided there were no good men in L.A., and went to sea as a ship's nurse in search of a husband.

"And I found one," she added coyly. "A musician in the cruise show."

She looked the picture of happiness, positively beamed as she told me her good fortune.

"I'm really happy for you, Connie. That's great!" I said. Right then, her good news made me happy too; a reminder of life's joys when I needed them most. Connie leaned toward me and lowered her voice.

"And this I never would have believed—he's Jewish! So my mom's delighted too!"

She gave me a hug, I wished her "mazel tov" with all my heart, and she disappeared to say hi to my mother. I was discharged the next day. Although the drain was still inside me, I felt a sense of my restored circulation; felt something powerful begin to stir in my consciousness, to which Dr. Castro's surgery opened the doors. There was a lot of pain where Dr. Ahn dislocated my shoulder, but none of it seemed to matter. Almost as soon as I woke, I sensed a desire, a need, to experience every moment of the recovery I felt sure was always possible when you can find the hidden path. Three days later, I saw Dr. Ahn to remove the drain.

"That must have been a very serious trauma you had," he commented. "Terrible mess. I've never seen such compression."

I recalled the doctors who missed the diagnosis completely.

"I don't know how much you'll recover," he continued, "but there'll be definite improvement from the surgery."

"Over what period of time?" I asked.

"You were so badly compressed for so long," Dr. Ahn reflected as he removed layers of surgical dressing. "Up to a year for your blood supply and nerves to resume normal shape and function, maybe another after that to get the full benefit."

True to his guarded optimism, my strength began to build in 2005. Everyone commented on it, including Dr. Duane McKay, the Leonardo da Vinci of dentists who realigned my jaw and rebalanced critical elements of my head and neck that enabled me to speak, chew, and smile. My appreciation for his success, and interest in his approach that made it possible, led to a great friendship, and in the spring, he invited me to a weekend conference in Milwaukee that showcased state-of-the-art technology for doctors of the head and neck.

At the BioResearch conference in Milwaukee, two hundred surgeons and specialists from around the world shared their secrets: cases which showed the limits of what they were taught in medical school and explained how they were forced to challenge conventional wisdom to heal their patients. Often, it seemed, it was no easier for doctors than it was for me to find the hidden path.

At the final reception, Duane made a point to introduce me to George Trachtenberg, a leading clinician from upstate New York, whose findings about the feet, posture, and gait were in publications ranging from *Bio-Mechanics* to *Podiatry Today*. When the reception ended, George carefully evaluated me as I weaved across the hotel banquet room, with the best shuffle I could. Every step took all my concentration, and my muscles never responded quite the same, so it amazed me when he saw a pattern.

"I watched the locators on your body, the defining skeletal markers," the gait expert explained.

"No one said I had a leg length discrepancy before," I said, as George very precisely marked up my brace.

"Ask your UCLA doctor to consider modifying this where I've indicated—to shorten the foot plate and add a heel lift."

On the return flight to L.A., I told Dr. McKay how I was writing a book to try to pass on information that might help people, and he enthusiastically described how these new technologies, and many of his insights gained through application of them, might be brought to more patients.

At the beginning of June, I was as ready as I ever would be for Dr. Endiman's next nerve block, to assess removal of my left rib. Far more crushed, to cut open the left side of my torso would be a lot more complex than the right, a lot more risky. As he conducted the test, my numbness dropped from eighty to twenty, and warmth spread into my left fingers again temporarily, after so long.

"When will you see your surgeon?" Endiman wrapped up quickly.

"In ten days, Doctor."

My next questions might have seemed strange in normal circumstances, but even if Ahn was so candid that the surgery Dr. Endiman just recommended might kill me, this might be my best chance to ask.

"After that surgery, can you check my pelvis and leg? Why do I have constant sciatic pain, and why can't I walk?"

No neurologist had come up with a complete answer, but then no one else diagnosed thoracic outlet until this team and its five-level data made it possible. Dr. Endiman was taken aback.

"Um, be happy to," he promised, "but one thing at a time!"

At his final consult for the second rib resection, Sam Ahn gave even more intense warnings of death and paralysis. He asked to see reports of all the earlier surgeries on my left shoulder, the area of his planned incision and extraction point.

"All your scars make it trickier. I'll book three hours, not two," was his worried conclusion, as he checked his calendar.

"Would it be good to allow more time to heal from my first rib extraction?" I tried.

I figured if it would improve my odds . . .

"About the same," he answered. It was up to me when I wanted to roll the dice.

"After eleven years, Doctor, I'd rather not wait any longer—whenever I can be your first operation of the day."

His assistant scheduled me for July 5. With Dr. Ahn having allocated more time, my check-in the day after the public holiday was even earlier, at 4:00 AM, so this time we left for Santa Monica-UCLA Medical Center well before dawn.

Feelgood hadn't called the night before, but we completed and faxed a questionnaire the hospital sent at the last minute straight back. One question asked the patient to "list your previous surgeries." By this point, mine ran three pages, single-spaced. When my parents and I compiled the list, the reminder of how many procedures I survived helped me face the surgery today. I'd accepted the possibility of death at Dr. Ahn's first surgery, and began the same meditation from the passenger seat of my mother's car as I gazed at the orange misty glow of streetlights drift by, carrying me closer.

There was no delay to check if my heart could tolerate removal of a second rib, because the hospital could rely on its successful removal of the first. So far, so good as, IV inserted on arrival, I was wheeled into pre-op. This time Feelgood was a genial older-looking man, a veteran of many years in the OR.

"Dr. Saxton said I should ask for the garbage anesthetic," I recited.

A kind, avuncular smile spread across Feelgood's face.

"And how do you spell that?" he asked.

Having achieved a Zen-like disassociation from life and acceptance of death, it was hard to be brought back.

"Er, g-a-r-b-a-g-e?"

"I'm not familiar with it."

Another avuncular smile that inspired confidence.

I tried my second request.

"Um, last time, the doctor said he'd leave something out so I'd be more lucid in the OR, but wouldn't throw up?"

"Oh, you don't want to be lucid in the OR. Not at all."

There followed the biggest avuncular smile yet.

It was Forrest Gump's box of chocolates. Whatever I did, I never knew whether the next chocolate out of it was a Feelgood, or a Feelbad, and this one hadn't a clue what I was talking about. At least he was punctual, when the rest of the team wasn't yet there. While we waited, I told him my case history, and felt even if I wouldn't receive the garbage cocktail, at least I had his interest. I focused on that crumb of comfort, and found the way back to inner balance. Finally, the head OR nurse arrived. Although the clock on the wall showed we were far behind schedule, she began to ask a series of preoperative questions. It dawned on me they were the same as the last-minute questionnaire we faxed the hospital the night before.

"So, why are you here today, Mr. Lewis?"

"Left ribectomy."

"And what other surgeries have you had?"

The last thing I could handle was to remind myself of them, but she waited for my answer. I looked at my nurse inquisitor, who stood by one of those carts on wheels hospitals use, and on which she doggedly wrote my answers on the file that would accompany me into the operating room. I craned my neck from my gurney and saw it.

"Look! There on top of my file—those three pages!"

Neatly single-spaced, it was our fax from the previous night.

"You have the list of all my surgeries—right there on top of your binder!" I said with triumphant relief.

The nurse hesitated, unsure of what to do. There was no way the list would fit on her form. At that moment, Ahn strode into pre-op, a captain on his deck.

"Good morning."

"Good morning, Dr. Ahn!" chorused his team,

physicians-in-training with the chance to observe and work under one of the country's top vascular surgeons.

They explained they still had to process my clinical history, and the OR nurse insisted she must review my surgeries, not all of which were familiar.

"The residents haven't evaluated him yet," she warned.

A moment's hesitation as he assessed, and then Dr. Ahn smiled slowly.

"Ready, Mr. Lewis?" he asked.

"I am."

"Get him into the OR," he told the nurse. "And I'll see you in there," he added to me.

The captain wasn't for waiting, and began his three-hour surgery to clear a second path of life-giving flow to a skull in which Dr. Castro had opened all the doors, to free the neurovascular supply to my brain.

I surfaced slowly into consciousness in the recovery room, and without the garbage anesthetic, threw up. A nurse placed a morphine button in my hand.

"Press whenever you need it," she said, and withdrew.

I lay awake all night, and listened to the sounds of the hospital, the sounds of life.

In the morning, a member of Dr. Ahn's team came to check on their patient. I thought she was the most radiant, beautiful woman I ever saw.

It gladdened my heart to see her after such a difficult night. She seemed especially interested in my chart. "Wow!" Doctor Radiant finally said. "You only pressed the pain button twice?"

Twice during the night my nervous system rebelled, threw my body into violent spasms. As brain and body struggled to consolidate the changes wrought inside, the morphine stopped the convulsions before I tore myself apart. She double checked the count and shook her head.

"How did the surgery go?" I asked.

"Dr. Ahn said you were one of the most challenging cases of his career," she confided, "and he's done hundreds and hundreds of these!" Then Doctor Radiant smiled and authorized my discharge.

In the days that followed, the panic attacks weren't gone, but the elephants moved far down the slope of consciousness to the crepuscular frontier between conscious and subconscious. It was as if I could feel my blood as it coursed through my veins and arteries. There was still unbelievable and unrelenting fatigue, only now it felt like the contented fatigue of a man who was years weary.

When I saw Dr. Ahn for follow-up, his nurse explained my pulse was down from eighty to sixty, which was closer to normal, but he frowned when he listened with his stethoscope and raised each arm.

"Yes, you've really good circulation now, except for your heart arrhythmia—that happens with your kind of chest injuries and compression." He sighed with regret, and confirmed I was in the care of a cardiologist as we shook farewell.

As August arrived, I realized that tinnitus, the nearly constant ringing in my ears every waking moment for the last eleven years, was now inconstant, and at times seemed almost completely gone. I felt calm, felt my mind was open.

Initiation crept back gradually, encouraged by Dr. Trachtenberg, the gait specialist I met in Milwaukee, with whom I began to correspond by e-mail, and who believed more could be done to advance my recovery. Also, I noticed for the first time how I never had stomach problems when I was in the hospital, but soon after discharge home, the bloating after meals began again. It occurred to me that I might ignore the recom-

mended special diets and drugs, and try to figure it out
for myself.

For the second half of September, I created an
identical morning routine, then changed only one item
at a time, and waited to see if it would be a good or bad
day. The answer was simple, yet perplexing. It wasn't
what I ate, because I had bad days when I ate nothing
at all until lunchtime. Nor was any specific exercise the
cause, whether Master Kim's intense home therapy, my
treadmill, or any other element of my daily home activities. But it was linked to exercise—any movement
in fact—and, in a strange way, to my clothes. When I
exercised in workout shorts—specifically, extra large
ones—I had a good day. If I chose to wear briefs, I had
a bad one. It was a deep nerve response that, once triggered, lasted the next two meals before my digestion
rebalanced. The response was near instant, and too low
on the slope to feel consciously. In the infinite analog
subtleties of our bodies, that stimulus alone sufficed.

I'd solved the problem simply, permanently, and
without medication. Not only was my nerve-blood circulation improved, but this step forward on the hidden
path meant that for the first time in years I digested
food properly, so my blood carried a fuller complement
of nutrition. If removal of the first rib started to awak-
en elements of my mind, removal of the second helped
them to coalesce.

It occurred to me I should start writing my book
to share some of the things I'd learned so far. I met my
former USC student Stu Pollard for lunch, who was
nearing distribution of his second feature. Having followed me through the years, he offered to take a look at
my manuscript when it was ready.

In October, as the benefits of Dr. Ahn's rib removal continued, I went to visit USC for the first time
since I left the campus eleven years earlier, an hour be-

fore the tragedy. I didn't feel physically or emotionally ready, but I needed a special computer and monitor for my vision if I was to try to write a book, develop projects, or produce movies and TV shows again. Thoughts about my future were often in my mind, it seemed.

Save for its pending name change to the School of Cinematic Arts in celebration of a record-breaking gift from the Lucasfilm Foundation, USC looked much the same as my mother drove us past the guard gate onto campus: the neat lawns and colorful flower beds, and the students headed to class. . . . I realized I still hadn't come to terms with the deficits and barriers that lay between me and full recovery. So much of my life was still in postponement, pending some final answers I was ever more determined to find.

The timing of the visit was forced on me in the best way, when USC's technology expert arranged a demonstration of the computer equipment I needed, and it was ready to view. It was another ray of hope when, in a mid-December letter, Victims of Crime approved my request for the ultra high-resolution monitor. A footnote to the dollars they authorized remarked, "This claim has now reached its maximum benefit of $46,000."

I relied on the Victims of Crime program as my insurer of last resort for critical medical bills, from Master Kim to Dr. McKay. With that exhausted, I now had only Medicare. But if it was the end of that road, it was the beginning of another.

 As 2006 arrived, my new computer, and ever improving blood-nerve circulation, enabled me to begin the first outline of this book.

CHAPTER TWENTY

WHERE TECHNOLOGY AND LIFE UNITE

*The sands of time were falling
From your fingers and your thumb,
And you were waiting
For the miracle,
For the miracle to come*
—Leonard Cohen,
"Waiting for the Miracle"

In the spring, I was encouraged further when Dr. McKay confirmed the long-term stability of my rebalanced jaw. There were no red dots involved in his treatment, and no fillings.

"Simon," he beamed at me in his clinic with a joyful enthusiasm second only to mine, "your teeth consistently hold your jaw in an adapted, functional alignment!"

Anything seemed possible if you made it to the right doctor, and in that frame of mind, I finally called the cell phone number Tova gave me two years before, when she swung through L.A. in her convertible.

"Is that really you?" she exclaimed from her home in San Francisco. "You come to the Jewish Federation's event next month in L.A., or else!"

There, I saw Jason, Tova's boyfriend, and the pair introduced me to their friends, a community into which I felt reborn.

"I'll be in touch again soon," I said at the end of the weekend, "when I'm back in action."

"Simon," she grinned happily, "you *are* back!"

But next morning, I suffered a massive, climactic crash. Days followed, stripped without warning out of my life. So soon after a social weekend gave me a glimpse of hope, the gap between how well Tova thought I was and how I felt inside remained untreated. The belief I had a worthwhile future was a delusion if no surgery or doctor could help, but Dr. Brodney gave me hope in one respect. Based on progress from his long-term vision treatment, he wrote a prescription that the "patient needs a driving evaluation," and I made an appointment at Cedars-Sinai to see whether there was any chance I could drive again.

I tried to prepare with games like *Midtown Madness* on my new computer. The driving simulations had little relevance to the real world outside my bedroom window, and as my mother watched my efforts to control a toy steering wheel, she feared the hospital would decide I was permanently unfit to drive. But the possibilities for me if I could regain mobility and function beckoned. With most of America I'd watched Howie Mandel host the premiere of *Deal or No Deal*, and to help build my confidence, my family took me to visit the soundstage for a taping.

The audience cheered as the hot models swept in with their briefcases, and in the blue room we met Howie and chatted. It was twelve years since he came into the Intensive Care Unit to offer comfort and help, and even if I was still disabled, Howie wanted me to understand that my friends were there for me, a reminder of the prize that awaited if I could follow the hidden path all the way to full recovery.

But I could not have felt less ready when I arrived at Cedars-Sinai's Outpatient Driving and Vision Program, and Erica, the nurse in charge, led me to a machine that looked like a fairground bumper car with steering wheel, brake, and accelerator pedals, but no wheels.

"Whenever those orange and green lights turn red, take your foot off the accelerator and brake as quick as you can," she explained.

A screen lit and played footage of a road from the driver's point of view. Through a mock windshield, it looked like I was driving my bumper car through rural America in the days of *American Graffiti*—the film was that old. When fin-tailed Oldsmobiles suddenly swerved into me, I had to turn away and brake. It was a simple and limited test that unnerved me.

"Your reflexes and crash avoidance skills are *acceptable*," reported Erica. Her tone made clear not to ask for details. "So we'll get you a one-day road permit, and evaluate whether you're safe to start lessons."

When we met the next day, my instructor was a middle-aged man with a penetrating gaze who saw his student's naked fear.

"Remember, this isn't the DMV . . . you're among friends!" Hank reassured me as we walked to a small red car parked outside. It felt surreal to shuffle to the driver's door, where Hank slid the seat all the way back for my left leg, encased in its hard plastic AFO shell, and then clumsily work my way in behind the wheel. Erica sat in back, laptop ready to take notes on this forty-eight-year-old novice, while Hank took the passenger seat with dual controls. I hesitantly laid one hand on the wheel, turned the key in the ignition with the other, and the engine hummed it was ready.

"Now, pull out," Hank said, quiet and firm, but I couldn't.

Hands frozen to the wheel, I stared at raindrops that began gently to speckle my windshield. We were on a side street behind a van and that's what Hank just told me to pull out from, but my mind felt no more capable of this than if I were under anesthetic in an operating room. At first nothing came to it from the past, from twenty years of driving, that made any more sense than if I simply closed my eyes as I did what he ordered.

"Mirror, signal, maneuver," I blurted suddenly, a teenage memory from England.

"The L.A. rule is SMOG," Hank corrected, while Erica noted my failure to comply from the backseat. "Signal, Mirror, Over the shoulder check . . . ," Hank whispered, "then *Go!*"

And after twelve years, that's what I jerkily tried, first on side roads with no traffic and then, on a sudden, we turned into the streaming humanity of Wilshire Boulevard. Hank occasionally operated the wipers so my white hands could stay clenched on the wheel.

"And now a left . . . and now we want to turn right." He sang the turns gently so as not to startle me, and observed my efforts.

Hank often took control, and explained how I must look down the road, anticipate problems ahead, and when the hour was up, his evaluation was that I should ask for a learner's permit.

"The DMV will test your vision and the rest pretty thoroughly," Hank warned as we parted.

I sent the Department of Motor Vehicles some forms, but it wasn't until our family barbecue on the Fourth of July that I felt a dizzying realization they meant I might drive again. My father, it turned out, also had news. By purest chance, he explained, one of his clients was newly married to a scientist who worked in medical research.

"Yesterday we were talking, and she asked how you were doing," my dad continued in his low key way, "and guess what? When I told her how you can't walk, she said she thinks her husband's working on that!"

"So I just reached Chuck at home," he smiled, to answer the question my whole family was about to ask, "and he told me his project not only has completed initial design, but the prototype's arrived from Israel, and you can go to the lab where he works and see it!"

That night, I checked the Web address my father gave me and learned of the Alfred Mann Foundation, a nonprofit medical research foundation focused on the development of implantable bionic technologies, from heart pacemakers to cochlear implants that restored hearing to thousands of deaf people, to research on an implantable eye sensor for the blind. This place, that none of my doctors told me about, where the impossible was being researched and developed, was a twenty-minute drive with my mother into the Santa Clarita Valley. The next day, with my father at work, my mother and I were on our way to see Chuck Byers, Senior Scientist of the Alfred Mann Foundation.

We drove past a guard gate and helicopter-landing pad into a park of landscaped gardens and terra cotta offices. Inside a pristine steel and glass research complex, Chuck guided us through state-of-the-art clean rooms, electron microscopes, and vacuum-sealed laser chambers; millions of dollars of equipment to build and test their latest generation BIONS. These bionic neurons were unlike anything I had ever seen before. Less than an inch long, the implantable titanium-tipped tubes could be monitored and controlled a hundred-times-a-second via radio signals, and were manufactured to function, networked inside the body, for over a hundred years.

"The goal is to restore function," Chuck explained. "One day, BIONS will detect a movement, calculate muscle length and limb acceleration, and then signal the other implanted microstimulators to complete it. About eighty percent of stroke patients have paralyzed limbs, and the BIONS will make it appear they've regained control of them."

He pointed to a wall chart of the human body, flecked with dozens of little tube icons, each a possible implant site. He smiled.

"Our goal one day is to link BIONS into the sensory cortex, so patients also have some sensation from their paralyzed limbs or prostheses."

After this vision of the future, Chuck brought us to a wood paneled conference room.

"Here's Ben," Chuck introduced an engineer in coat and tie who joined us there, "to show you what we're working on now. He's come from Israel to oversee the U.S. introduction of our Neurological Electrical Stimulation System, NESS for short."

Ben very formally took out a small device labeled H200. The "h" stood for "hand," Chuck explained, and Ben wrapped it around his forearm, showing how the NESS restored function to fingers and wrists. After the promise of Chuck's tour, I couldn't help my disappointment.

"I'm sorry, it's my leg that needs help," I explained, "I can't walk."

I rolled up my pant leg and showed them the heavy plastic brace up to my knee, with protective socks pulled over the top. It was painfully hot and uncomfortable year round, but especially so when it was over a hundred degrees outside, like today. Ben carefully set a small canvas travel bag on the table.

"You have tendon surgery?" he quizzed in a

strong, perhaps originally Russian, accent.

If that ruled me out for whatever was in the bag, I was doubly grateful I never followed the recommendation of Rancho Los Amigos and other clinics, but waited for something better to come along.

"No," I said, and held my breath as Ben unzipped the bag.

"This is new L300, for leg," he announced proudly, and then set a small blue-gray device that looked like an athlete's knee guard on the table.

I remembered the functional stimulation unit at Cedars-Sinai that restored use of my left arm. In spite of many efforts since, I never found a therapist who would use it to bring back my left leg the same way. The bulky device required a shoulder sling to carry, and at any attempt to walk, its electrodes promptly fell off. The NESS looked like a prayer come true. Single-handedly attachable for patients with use of only one limb, it clipped easily onto the calf. Inside, were two pre-positioned electrodes.

"Whenever I thought about how long I practiced something when I was a baby to learn it," I said, "it seemed to me twenty minutes of physical therapy couldn't come close. This device could send the right message thousands of times."

"That's the concept," Chuck nodded. "In our lab tests, we saw some retraining of the brain, some memory of muscle sequences that we programmed into the NESS, but we don't know the extent."

"After two months, the effects, they fade away. So far . . . ," Ben added cautiously. So much remained unknown to the scientists in the room.

"We understand," my mother struggled to contain her hopes, focused not on distant research, but the potential lightning in a box that sat on the table in front of us.

"How does Simon get one?"

Mr. Rubin, an executive from marketing and customer service, joined us to explain that, with the NESS prototype and its engineer arrived, they could start beta trials to seek FDA approval.

"I can take Simon wherever you say," my mother offered. Mr. Rubin explained that if the NESS received FDA approval, Bioness would market the technology to rehab facilities, and train their therapists on proper use of the equipment.

"And how much would it cost?" I asked nervously.

"Until we hear from the FDA we won't price it," he shrugged. "The hand device is $6,000, so likely in that range, and we help patients to apply for insurance coverage."

"No. Not necessary shave legs," Ben laughed at my next question. Unlike the electrodes on other medical devices, the NESS held them firmly enough to make even that discomfort unnecessary. It seemed perfectly designed in every respect.

"Yesterday, I use for whole day," Ben grinned as he bent down and swiftly put on the little device to demonstrate. He took the NESS off with equal ease, smiled with pride, and handed it to us for a closer look. It was less than four inches wide, and made of a material designed to let the skin breathe. This meant the suffocating hard plastic of my brace and the protective sock up to my knee might be things of the past; that I could once again wear socks the same length, and walk in shorts without people staring as I struggled with every step.

Ben and Chuck demonstrated how the NESS worked by a pressure sensor under the insole, which triggered as the wearer's heel left the ground. A small transmitter clipped to the shoe relayed data up to the NESS.

"When can I get one?" I asked, the device in my hand.

"Depends on FDA approval, and that's anyone's guess. But keep in touch," Mr. Rubin invited brightly, "and track our progress!"

A sense of the wind at my back once more, my mother took me to the Van Nuys DMV office the next week. My application form with Hank's upbeat evaluation at the Cedars driving program had brought a Notice of Interview before an officer at the DMV's Safety Office, reserved for special vehicles and the disabled.

"A written test is required as part of this interview," it warned, not that anyone at Cedars told me to prepare for one, but my hearing officer gave me positive news.

"You passed the written test. Well done, Mr. Lewis!" she congratulated. With such a good start, I was eager for my friendly officer's advice on the best driving school to turn theory into practice.

"Thank you." I began. "Can you recommend—"

"Please wait." She put finger to her lips for silence. "Now raise your right hand."

She waited until I complied, then activated a digital recorder on her desk.

"Mr. Lewis, do you swear to tell the truth, the whole truth, and nothing but the truth, so help you God?"

I wanted to finish my question, but my officer seemed to have started some kind of trial, at the end of which she would rule on my application for driving lessons. I tried to figure out what to say to make her switch off the recorder, but the only reply I could think of was, "Yes . . . I swear."

Nor was there a chance to speak as she recited admission into evidence of various "exhibits" I had never seen before, which she dropped into the DMV's permanent record on me. The machinery of state government in gear, she began the trial that would determine her decision, and my driving future.

"Now, Mr. Lewis," she opened, "is it your sworn testimony that as of today you are safe on the road, and ready to take the State of California driving test?"

I watched the red blinking light on her digital recorder, tried to figure out what to say to fill the ominous silence, and furiously wondered what someone hadn't told me this time.

"Um, I think I'd like some lessons first."

I tried to sound rational; that after twelve years, this was my strategy, and hoped she would turn nice again and tell me what to do. Instead, her face hardened as she shut off the recorder, my hearing over before it began. As we parted, my officer explained I was supposed to contact the DMV only after something called "an occupational therapy driving program" certified I was ready.

The setback made me yearn for mobility all the more. That week, while I researched driving programs, I saw my internist Dr. Brousseau and discussed the conflicting diagnoses over the last twelve years, and why I must see Dr. Endiman, the star neurologist, for his promised test on my left leg so I could walk again.

"I don't want to disappoint you, Simon," Brousseau said, "but I've had other patients who were turned down." His stethoscope in play, he continued to lean over intently, head bowed to my chest.

"I agree with Dr. Ahn," he frowned. "We need to do a regular Holter test to check your heart. There are pauses when it doesn't beat." He concluded his examination and shook my hand. "Maybe you're used to that, but it makes me nervous!"

It didn't seem the right time to tell my doctor what made me nervous—the imminent start of driving lessons at the closest program, offered by a facility I knew well. On the fourth floor of Northridge Hospital Medical Center was the office of Gayle San Marco, coordinator of its Driver Preparation program, and when he arrived, Ken proved to be a therapist-turned-instructor with blond hair, clear blue eyes, and a deep calm voice.

"We'll help you if we can," he encouraged, and assisted me into the hospital's specially adapted car, loaded with mirrors in every direction and a warning sign on the roof so big it looked like a sail. To begin his evaluation, he eased the dual control vehicle off the hospital grounds and turned past the TGIC brain injury rehabilitation house, still well maintained, with a new, longer ramp up to the front door where Ola first greeted me so many years before. After a short route along quiet side streets, Ken reported that it would take at least seven more sessions, culminating with Gayle's evaluation from the backseat to determine whether I could safely attempt to drive.

With that underway, I called Eric Weissmann, a leading entertainment attorney and senior partner of his Beverly Hills law firm. It was the first time I had called him in over twelve years, but Eric invited me for lunch the next day, our friendship unchanged. At lunch, I gave him the first chapters of my manuscript, and that week I also wore another Holter heart monitor as Dr. Brousseau prescribed. But my unwavering attention was fixed on my Friday morning appointment with Dr. Endiman, the star neurologist. I tried not to let my hopes rise when he entered our cubicle at his clinic, about to finish a Snickers bar.

I explained how the removal of my ribs helped after his successful nerve blocks, but Dr. Endiman wasn't interested in the past as he watched me walk about the room, checked my chart, and couldn't remember the tests he promised. But he had another answer for my leg, and could treat me with no more tests or surgery.

"It's very clear," he diagnosed, "your muscles don't release—and that's from brain injury."

For the fatigue this caused, he prescribed Provigil, a stimulant used by the military, and to recover use of my leg, a lifelong series of Botox injections, the kind that the neurologist in Scottsdale, mentioned.

"Are there risks with Botox?" I asked, as I tried to remember the advice at the Arizona Dystonia Institute.

"Yes, but I use the smallest amount," Dr. Endiman assured. "And I do it guided by both an EMG and ultrasound, so it goes exactly where needed with pinpoint accuracy."

"Have you treated people like Simon who've suffered both stroke and brain injury?" asked my mother.

"Thousands," he replied, "and it's my precision in targeting that makes the difference between success and failure."

I thought of Rancho Los Amigos and the guru of gait, and their recommendation of multiple tendon transfer surgeries.

"I don't think anyone does those any more, do they?" Dr. Endiman smiled back.

My family and I struggled through the weekend with whether to wait on FDA approval of the NESS, a process that might take years, or be treated immediately by a specialist who promised to use new technology and, within minutes, enable me to walk again. The wait for a miracle to come along, in the form of Endiman's new technology, already consumed most of the year. By Sunday night, my family agreed: It was time to commit to Dr. Endiman's lifelong rehabilitation with Botox shots, and we faxed my treatment consent form to his clinic.

On Monday morning, the phone rang. It was Dr. Endiman's sympathetic office manager.

"I'm sorry to advise you, Mr. Lewis, that UCLA Medical Group has already declined your consultation at this clinic," she opened, her voice low with frustration. "Under no circumstances will UCLA reimburse any treatment by Dr. Endiman."

It was vital that insurance pay so I could afford Botox injections and walk for the rest of my life, so we drove straight over to UCLA, determined to make it happen.

We headed anxiously into the UCLA neurology department, and ran into Dr. Saxton in the front lobby, busy but pleased to see us.

"I've just added Saturday clinics!" she said, so we could see her that week, which alone made our trip worthwhile, and Dolly thought Botox sounded like a very good idea, before she pressed on to her patient. As we entered the reception in search of someone to reverse our latest insurance denial, by chance Dr. Collins was at the counter. His face lit with a broad smile.

"Lewis!" he exclaimed. "And where's your mother?"

"Right here, as usual!" she chimed in.

"Dr. Collins," I seized the chance and jumped right to my question, "what do you think of Botox?"

"For you? *Very bad idea*. Ask Dolly. She'll tell you why."

"But just now she told me it could help." I felt awkward, but he was unfazed.

"Botox damages nerves. It persists in our system, so it keeps damaging them. You'll lose what little control you've got of your leg, Lewis, until you have nothing!"

I repeated Dr. Endiman's description of how he used an EMG and an ultrasound for guidance to assure success. Dr. Collins didn't answer.

"I guess you've told me your medical opinion," I said, confused as to whose advice to follow. He smiled kindly and looked into my eyes. "All your problems are circulatory," he said.

"Well, the rib resections made a big difference," I thanked him. Of that, at least, I was sure.

"That's what we like to hear!" he retorted. As his pager called him away, he turned back.

"You *saw* Dolly?" he asked, as it dawned on him that I mentioned her.

"Which way did she go? Which way?!" he asked urgently.

I pointed, and he was gone.

My mother and I returned for Dr. Saxton's Saturday clinic. I explained how, given Dr. Collins's warning, I put Dr. Endiman's Botox shots on hold for however long FDA approval of the NESS might take. I told Dolly how much better I grasped and acted on what people said. Things, it seemed, became clearer almost day by day.

"It's changed Simon so much," my mother agreed. "Thank you, as only a mother can, for bringing back my son!"

"Oh . . . we just did our job, that's all," Dolly smiled. "And Simon, I don't think you need Provigil. Your energy is way up!"

"I've just started to feel that," I answered reflexively, and was surprised in that moment to realize both that I thought what Dolly said was true, and emotionally felt it. I felt the gap, which I described as a broken yardstick to Dr. Whitney at Cedars almost thirteen years before and ever since, begin to *connect*, to the point I could assess my mind.

"Simon," Dr. Saxton reassured, "you've come a long way, and you'll go a lot further. Our bodies are wonderful, they regenerate all the time."

"When you have the right doctors," I replied, as we left.

There were other reasons to be grateful. In October, on the eve of the Day of Atonement, the holiest night of the Jewish calendar, my niece Nikki sang the *Kol Nidre* prayer, her great voice resonating through the temple's congregation and our entire family. An ancient Aramaic phrase, the prayer annuls our empty vows to God and frees us to go into our future. We were all there. David and Lilly's son Jason, now an undergrad at Indiana University's business program, and on the college water polo team. But in his cupboard at home, he still kept Otto, the stuffed toy duck he dragged into my hospital room at Cedars when he was six. There was Stephanie, at the end of her junior year at NYU, Jonathan and Elinor with their toddlers Sammy and Rachel, and my parents, hopeful once again the new year might bring answers.

As 2007 began, Steve Wasserman, a literary agent in New York to whom I submitted a draft of my book, confirmed that he would represent me and try to find a publisher to tell my story of recovery. Then I called Mr. Rubin at Bioness headquarters, to check on progress with the NESS.

"Your timing's perfect!" he exclaimed, and then stopped short.

"Simon, you, don't have any metal hardware in your body, do you?"

Patients with electrical or metallic implants, he explained, weren't eligible as first users of the NESS. I thanked God and my surgeons that no titanium remained.

"Not any more."

"Well in that case, I can tell you we expect FDA approval any day!"

As soon as it came through, Mr. Rubin sent one of the first NESS L300s by messenger, and the next morning my mother drove me and the unopened box to Casa

Colina Rehabilitation Center in Pomona. An hour from our home, Casa Colina was a beautiful Spanish-styled campus dotted with pine trees, dedicated to the rehabilitation of patients at every level of trauma and disability.

In the gym, fully equipped with the most advanced computerized test systems available, I met Mathu Hanson, head neurological therapist. We shook hands and he began to program the NESS's control unit. I'd give anything to qualify for it, but under the watchful gaze of Steven Ulrich, Bioness's Regional Clinical Specialist, who in turn was under FDA oversight, I knew that depended on Mathu's evaluation. The one-hour session turned to nearly two, so much was at stake with this fantastic device, which could deliver electrical pulses timed to my footsteps.

Once the NESS was calibrated, Mathu took me outside to a test track around a small grass lawn for my first effort to walk solo, with no brace, no cane, and with no support other than hope and this device.

"You first did this when you were two," Mathu encouraged, "and back then it wasn't something you thought about, you just woke up one day and did it."

Ever since, I realized, I never thought about walking or picking up my feet with each step. The precious sequence, wired into our subconscious before birth, worked right up to my crash, and none of my efforts ever since could reach that community of nerve paths. I realized my whole body was tense with fear.

"Don't think. Don't try. . . . *Walk*," Mathu urged.

And when I didn't think, when I let the NESS take over control of my leg, for the first time in thirteen years I took my first normal steps.

By the end, Mathu confirmed I was eligible, and the Bioness sales department began paperwork for me to buy a NESS, and seek insurance coverage for it. Mathu took the entire next session to experiment. I felt current flow, activate muscles in perfect time and sequence, and looked over to my hero.

"I'm dialing it up as safely as I can!" Mathu whispered to preserve a professional atmosphere in the gym. There was no way to know if my damaged brain could learn how to trigger correct sequences again, but it would be one of the first to get this chance.

Mathu explained the conditioning protocol to acclimate my system. By the end of a month, if all went well, I'd wear my NESS all day. The user's guide made no promises. It warned that "the long-term effects of chronic electrical stimulation are unknown," but its short-term effects were clear. In my hard plastic brace, I never managed more on a treadmill with my cane than a snail's pace of half a mile an hour.

With the NESS, the next morning I pressed the speed button until it doubled. By the third session at Casa, the NESS changed my view of the world; I looked up when I walked, and took in more of my surroundings. If I ignored the persistent sciatic pain that crept in, I could walk two thirty-minute sessions at the higher speed.

"I was skeptical about this device when they called," Mathu confided. He was trained to immobilize and brace the weakened limbs of stroke- and head-injured patients. Before the NESS, that was the only treatment available. With a personal mounting interest as he refined settings, Mathu found the optimum placement, the neurological sweet spot.

"Simon," he exclaimed with excitement, "you're walking naturally!"

From time to time, Bioness's representative Steven visited to record the first patient experiences with a NESS. He seemed very interested in mine, confirmed when he relayed a company request to film me in a news release. By week three, my speed quadrupled as the NESS algorithms tracked my gait, improved my balance, and made me more confident to go out in the community. By the end of the month, my use of the NESS totaled over seventy hours, over three constant days of targeted functional stimulation; more than the previous thirteen years combined. Every muscle in my left leg grew in strength by a full point in the therapists' 0–5 scale that Mathu used to evaluate them, where each increase in the degree of strength correlates to a degree of increase in capacity to function. Mathu was stunned by the change.

"It makes sense to bring you here for a second month and increase sessions to twice a week, see how far we can bring your pelvis back," he explained, as he wrote an authorization and set a new goal. "So, let's see what we can do!"

Linda, Bioness's marketing liaison, filmed me walking normally across the gym, then outside in the open with my mother, also a star for the day. It took no acting skill to look as happy as we felt. Bioness uplinked the story by satellite to news bureaus, and it went so well that an invitation came for KABC-TV to interview me.

"If you take charge and think long-term, you can accomplish miraculous things," I said in the story ABC aired on the evening news. Invited back to the Mann Foundation campus, I saw the two-story Bioness headquarters under construction, and met Alfred Mann himself, a youthful octogenarian who still ran a dozen companies and worked as many hours a day, with his equally energetic wife. Along with other first users who found their way from neurological trauma to the NESS, Bioness asked if we would participate in media outreach to help others.

The NESS user guide emphatically warned that

it could not be used with any hard conventional shoe orthotics, since they might break the pressure sensor on which the system depended, and Dr. Trachtenberg offered his expertise to help overcome this challenge. A friend since Dr. McKay introduced us in Milwaukee, he began a research project to see if he could redesign his protocols to combine both systems. Bioness shipped the materials he needed from Israel to his clinic, and Dr. Trachtenberg went to work.

There was progress, too, in L.A. After many months of driving lessons, with big smiles Gayle and Ken said I was ready for my road test. I felt physically prepared, too. At Casa Colina, Mathu had ramped up my program and confided this increased level of activity was "something I normally only give to athletes." If the Northridge clearance meant I was ready to drive, the NESS made me confident I could walk to my destination from wherever I parked.

Everything was on track when the day in March arrived, and I drove with Ken to the Van Nuys Department of Motor Vehicles for my test. Mr. Harvey arrived punctually. From behind owlish horn-rimmed glasses, my soft-spoken driving examiner looked and sounded like a man who made no ripples at the DMV during many years of service.

"I understand you were injured," Harvey commented kindly from the passenger side as I climbed awkwardly behind the wheel. "I won't give any instruction intended to confuse or mislead you."

He enunciated every word slowly for my benefit and I felt reassured, if a little patronized.

"Good luck!" he finished with a little smile, as I began, carefully scanning every intersection as instructed, and followed Harvey's instructions, given so quietly they were barely audible over the engine. Twice, he spun around to look behind our car, and then scribbled notes. Ken told me in advance to ignore this, so all was well. I knew I was home free when Harvey instructed me to turn left. The Van Nuys DMV office, and Ken, waited for me fifty yards up that road.

After my light turned green and I advanced into the intersection, a pedestrian hurried into the crosswalk. As I noticed her and slowed, Harvey found his voice.

"*What happened there*?!" he shouted, as he seized hold of the wheel and floored the brake. I was too shaken to answer, any confidence shattered by my examiner's belief I endangered a pedestrian. Whatever I said couldn't change the outcome; once the examiner intervened, my test was over. I watched the pedestrian clear the crosswalk a second later, and made the turn.

"I know what I'd do if this was a regular test," Harvey resumed his soft tone as we pulled into the DMV parking lot, "but that's up to Driver Safety."

Ken walked over to join us, neutral professionals as Harvey showed his notes, then left.

"I don't think I did anything wrong," I sighed on our way back to Northridge, "but I guess the examiner's the final word." It made no sense to continue if, after months of lessons, the expert thought I was a danger to others.

"I couldn't believe it when Harvey changed direction at the DMV and walked up to us," Ken fumed by way of reply.

"You recognized him?"

"Yeah, hadn't seen him for over a year and thought he must'a fallen off the face of the Earth," Ken mused. "Care to guess, Simon, in the twelve years I've been helping clients with disabilities learn to drive, how many he's passed?"

"Less than half?" I guessed from Ken's frustration.

"No, Simon, you'd have been the first!"

On his formal written report, my pit bull examiner not only failed me, but also certified I would not benefit from further lessons, and that the California DMV should never let me take the test again. I knew how to overcome arbitrary rejection by insurers, but this was the first by the government. To help my appeal, Northridge Hospital wrote to the DMV and requested a special hearing, while I threw myself into the Casa program. By this point, with the NESS activated, I could hold a punching bag high, then kick-box at Mathu's therapy trainee, as he circled.

"Move your feet so your pelvis faces toward where you need to kick," Mathu urged. I kicked as hard as I could, tears of sweat and frustration in my eyes.

I still had constant sciatic pain, but George's research with the materials sent by the NESS company from Israel was complete. Since my niece Stephanie was about to graduate from NYU and my family planned to join her in Manhattan to celebrate, it was the perfect time to visit Dr. Trachtenberg's clinic and put his ideas into practice.

In New York, I also reunited with my friend, director and film professor David Irving, to talk about a movie he wanted me to produce. The NESS gave me the freedom to walk from our hotel to lunch with the film's writer without thinking about every step. Save for my sciatic pain, it was mobility easier than I ever dreamed possible.

The Stars and Stripes waved in the breezy sunshine as an early morning car drove me through the small college town of Vestal, to rendezvous with Dr. Trachtenberg at a local specialist, whose pelvic X-ray showed my right leg was shorter, and confirmed George's visual assessment in Milwaukee.

"And," he sighed, "that was when you wore a brace, which added a third of an inch to your left leg."

We went on to George's clinic, one of few private facilities in the country dedicated to computerized and video analysis of walking, where I stood for the first time in the gait studio I saw on his website. George devoted the whole day to my evaluation, as assistants used magic marker points on knee, calf, and ankle—back, front, and side—for visual reference, slated the shot, and began the unique series of tests for my experimental case, in the order he prescribed.

"I've got four cameras on you to compare your alignment from front, back, and both sides," my friend the foot surgeon explained, as his technicians downloaded data. "So if something's wrong in one view, I can correlate it to the rest of your body and posture."

"And the pads in my shoes?"

"Sensors that give me up to fifty thousand pieces of information. Think of this as if I'm doing an EKG of your feet; as if I can see inside your shoes while you're walking."

Graphic indications of time, force, and pressure, appeared on George's monitors, tied to the position of ankle and foot, measured sixty-times-a-second.

As the day advanced, he took two sets of impressions, one pair to be worn with the NESS and the other without, so I would be prepared for whatever the future held. Each step sought for the highest accuracy and quality, to the extent that one impression was discarded because the resin was flawed.

"Perhaps there was a pinhole and some air got to it," he muttered as he handed off the cast and started over. He approached his data differently than a researcher because his treatment philosophy was different.

"Some of what I do is based on intuition," he offered. "An F-Scan can't give answers on its own. I need the X-rays, video, and computer data, then form an impression from what they indicate," he explained, his focus on the images on multiple monitors. "The technology is how I make an exact comparison before and after I prescribe orthotics that optimize your gait," he smiled as he saw me into a car back to New York, and assistants sent the casts to his custom orthotics manufacturer. And on Friday when I returned to pick them up, they felt different from anything I put in my shoes before.

"They're supposed to," he laughed with delight.

The NESS worked fine with them. As we walked around outside George's clinic, he explained how I must retrain my posture, and look up to the horizon. And back in Manhattan toward the end of our trip, as I walked with my parents through the Museum of Modern Art and looked up at the pictures, I found I could think about them, not my feet. When I woke next morning, the time of maximum sciatic pain for so many years, there was none. George's orthotics, that optimally balanced my legs and gait, had relieved it.

During my family's last morning in New York, my cousin Richard joined us for breakfast. Richard grew up in London like me, but before he moved to Manhattan, he lived in Israel for many years and spoke fluent Hebrew. I demonstrated how easily I could walk around the restaurant, and then rolled up my pant leg to show Richard the fantastic Israeli device that made it possible.

"Here's my NESS, short for Neurological Electrical Stimulation System," I recited happily. Richard reacted to the logo.

"Simon, you do know what 'ness' means in Hebrew, right?"

"Afraid not," I confessed.

My cousin smiled.

"It means 'miracle.'"

CHAPTER TWENTY-ONE

FULL RECOVERY: MIND, BODY, AND SOUL

He who saves a single life,
saves the entire world
—Sanhedrin 4:9

At Casa Colina, the exercises Mathu improvised reached new levels. He set up a beam, three inches wide, and sloped it at an angle so that as I put all my weight on my weak leg and worked backwards, the beam got higher and harder for me to clear with my other leg.

"Now, step up."

With assistance from Mathu and his intern, I wobbled up onto the narrow beam at its highest point. Mathu gestured to pull up a small stool on wheels. "Now, right foot on that stool, Simon, and draw an arc with it from left to right, and back." Assisted by the NESS, I maintained balance and, gradually, inched the stool in a curve around me.

"Look," Mathu tapped his control unit at the end of the session, "your first day here you walked nineteen steps with the NESS. As of today . . ." His stylus scrolled through my record at Casa Colina. "You've walked . . . 321,561."

"That sounds pretty good," I said.

"Your progress is remarkable," Mathu answered quietly as he double-checked his timings, then looked up. "Now let's build your pelvis strength, until, Simon," he paused, "you can bronze your cane!"

I might be free of it at last.

When Tova's wedding invitation arrived in the mail, I knew it was the right time to confront another barrier. The marriage to Jason, Tova's boyfriend since Jewish camp, would be in San Francisco. The independence I felt walking around Manhattan, and memory of Tova's overnight flight from Rome to join Marcy for our wedding, made me determined to make it to Tova's.

Repeated follow-up calls secured the new DMV hearing requested by Gayle on behalf of Northridge Hospital's Driver Preparation program. Once we were on the record, she submitted her request for the DMV to override Harvey's decision.

"Right now I can only afford one lesson a week at the hospital. I need more time behind the wheel," I pleaded. Gayle explained how seriously the hospital took its responsibility to submit only qualified drivers to the DMV, the terrible loss of freedom to deny qualified clients, elderly and disabled alike, their license.

My hearing officer listened without comment.

"When I looked at your file I asked myself, 'What does Simon Lewis want?'" she said after a long silence. It was a fair question.

"I figured . . . probably another test and a permit for more lessons," she answered herself evenly. Then she beamed at us, another fair public servant who wanted to help, and gave me everything I asked.

Able to use any instructor over twenty-five, we found Bryan Burrage, a professional driver and expert instructor. With a discipline honed in college football plays and the Air Force, Bryan offered a perfect precision-driving program. We drove two hours at a time in his dual-control instructor's car, as Bryan drilled me on professional, hand-over-hand steering. The DMV office in Arleta had wider streets, I learned, and fewer pedestrians than my first test in Van Nuys where my examiner intervened on my last turn. With my parents' help, in readiness for the wedding I sold my stick-shift convertible, bought their four-door automatic, and practiced every day for the freeway drive to San Francisco.

In August, my assigned examiner at the Arleta DMV, clipboard in hand, climbed into the passenger seat of Bryan's car with me at the wheel. Without a word, Bryan waved us goodbye, and I followed Gloria's instructions as I drove the dual-control car out the parking lot onto a side street, turned right again, and took the first right, which brought us back onto the main boulevard in front of the DMV.

"Will you drive the freeway today?" Gloria asked, as I knew she would, and visions of the open road to San Francisco beckoned.

"Yes, thank you . . . ," I began, then focused on a homeless man, who in the middle of this commercial city block, worked a supermarket grocery cart filled with all his possessions across four lanes of fast traffic. To warn the driver behind me, who wouldn't expect a sudden stop in a business zone, I feathered the brakes at first, to flash my taillights.

"You're stopping, right?" Gloria quizzed.

I breathed in to answer.

"I—"

Gloria hit the brakes.

"Am . . ."

The homeless man crossed safely in front.

"Turn back into the parking lot," Gloria continued as she scribbled notes, the test over so fast Bryan was still there.

"Candidate accelerated toward a pedestrian," Gloria explained, and showed her written report: "Pedestrian was crossing street and applicant made no attempt to slow down. Examiner told applicant to slow down and stepped on brakes."

"I *was* braking!" I gasped, dreams of San Francisco exposed as fantasy, my confidence broken when the expert said I almost killed a homeless man. Bryan saw it.

"If Mr. Lewis accelerated, that means his foot was on the *gas*," he said, "and you were right to fail him. But if he was slowing, like he says, then his foot was on the *brake*. So where was his foot?"

Bryan stared hard at the examiner, who said nothing. I learned later that the DMV, through budget cuts, axed its specially trained examiners for elderly and challenged drivers, who knew how to assess them for road awareness and safety.

"You drive the route hundreds of times," Bryan's anger rose through her silence, "if it's a race for the brake pedal, the disabled don't stand a chance!"

"It's no big deal," Gloria wavered. "It's his first attempt and I wrote that he should take it a second time."

My dedicated instructor lost it.

"No . . . no . . . *no* . . . ," he groaned. "Didn't you check his paperwork? This *was* his second. One more fail—and he's done!"

When I called Tova's home number to make my apologies, a small voice I barely recognized as hers picked up. The wedding was off. Jason had backed out of their marriage.

"All the out-of-towners have left," she sobbed, "but I have a spare room, so *please* come meet my friends."

I couldn't let her down, but felt unable to undertake such a journey alone. My best friend Dave the director volunteered, happy to help me navigate the airports and see me into a cab to Tova's address, while he spent the weekend with a girlfriend who also lived in San Francisco.

Tova was relieved to see me. Overwhelmed with advice from her friends and family, determined to follow some of it and meet new people, she took me to the Redwood Room at the Clift Hotel the evening I arrived. Because of my NESS, I could walk through the packed nightclub and look up at digital portraits on plasma monitors, of people whose eyes looked back, and followed mine. Tova left for the restroom, and when she made it back through a room full of men on the pull, she wore a baseball cap given to her by a guy her parents might wish for her: the perfect trifecta of young, Jewish, and attorney. David was handsome, too, and out for his last night in San Francisco after a tour of the wine country with his buddy, who was drunk and stalled by the bar. As we chatted, David slid his hand nonchalantly inside the back of Tova's jeans, detectable only from her deep red flush.

"I need to know why I want to kiss a boy," she sighed as we left him at the bar, "and I know I belong with Jason."

She looked up at me, a deserted bride uncertain of her future.

The following evening, the last of my trip, we headed to an Italian restaurant in North Beach with a pair of Tova's closest friends. Joey was a successful commercial insurance broker. Early thirties, bald, and buff, he was with Lisa, who came to San Francisco to open the workout gym where they met. A network producer had selected Joey for the pilot of a reality dating show, with love coaches to tell girls how to get their guy and find true love, and the guys how to behave. You could see why they cast Joey. His all-black SUV surged through the night, subwoofers at full blast. Lisa complained.

"Too loud for you, buddy?!" Joey roared over his shoulder as we crested over one of San Francisco's hills. I could feel my remaining ribs vibrate, resonate, and throb to the beat.

"It's great, Joey."

This trip with Tova and her friends made everything better than great. Joey took it well.

"You are a man who embraces life," he enunciated through his thick New Jersey accent, and grasped my hand intently before he negotiated the next crest perfectly, just shy of takeoff. At the restaurant, Joey ordered two bottles of their finest red, and as we chatted over our meal, Tova revealed how, with persuasion from her parents, she reluctantly signed onto JDate, the Jewish online dating service. The first contact she braced herself to meet for tea the next day was, she smiled, a Jewish Englishman named Simon.

"I don't believe it!" Joey roared as he ordered espresso and Amaretto shots for the table, shaken by more than the name coincidence. In the anonymous, first-name-only world of online dating, English Simon with a BMW bike was Joey's assistant. San Francisco, it turned out, really was a small town.

"He's a good man, Tova. Best assistant I ever had!" he exclaimed. As more wine flowed, we talked about Tova's love for Jason, about Marcy and me; about my book to help others, which Steve, my agent, would send to publishers and my former student wanted to adapt into a movie; and about our futures. Over dessert, Lisa had a special gift for me that she made by hand: an amulet, with five linked beads of intricate design.

"It's a hamsa," she explained, a symbol shared by Jews and Muslims alike; an ancient belief that predates both religions.

"I thought of you, Simon, because you hang it near you," she added, "to ward off the evil eye and keep demons at bay."

I thought of the protecting hands that brought me through the last years, and thanked her for the amulet. When our check arrived, Joey refused to let me pay.

"You will never buy me a meal," he declared as we left the restaurant. He held me in a tight bear hug. "But you always gotta buy the next guy's."

Down the block, we strolled into a mojito bar for a final nightcap, and another soda for me. As the live salsa group performed onstage, its lead singer worked through the room and brought us onto the dance floor, to the Caribbean rhythm and his rich baritone voice.

With the newfound mobility of my NESS, I managed to dance with Tova, Joey, and Lisa, hip to hip amongst the crowd, swaying to the intoxicating beat.

"I can't believe how much you've improved since I last saw you," Tova said and smiled softly, subdued. I remembered the joyful, energized young woman who flew from a consulting job in Italy to my wedding.

"I guess we're both survivors, Tova . . . right?"

We hugged, a moment passed between us, until I saw how conflicted she was, not reconciled with her lost fiancé.

"We have to make the most of every chance, Tova, every day we get."

"And how about you, Simon?" she pressed, her eyes tearful with the same question, "Are you ready for your future?"

And for the first time in that North Beach mojito bar, I felt close to an answer.

"Now, why don't you go ask that woman to dance?" Tova challenged, and without my cane I walked over to the bar.

Lindsay took a fresh drink with her before we headed toward the dance floor, where she stumbled against me and spilled some.

"You're not leaving soon?" I asked.

"What's it to you?" My dance partner narrowed her eyes.

"You might need some time before you get behind the wheel," I said. It was awkward, but true.

"Simon . . . screw you," she retorted thickly, and shook me off.

As Tova and her friends rejoined me, she eyed me curiously. "You look crazy happy, but your first dance never made it to the floor."

"She told me to go to hell," I nodded.

"And that's good?"

"Yes, I guess I annoyed her."

"Right, Sherlock," Tova smiled, "I didn't know you could read minds. Maybe you could do that for my fiancé. Anyway, you are crazy if you think that went well."

"But it did," I replied, as it dawned on me why my dance partner's instant rejection was a complete success.

"Tova, have you ever been rude to someone in a wheelchair?"

"Can't say I have," she said, swaying with me to the melody.

"Even if they just ran over your toes?" I continued. "And why's that?"

"Because," Tova began, "you're supposed to be nice to people less fortunate, with disabilities. . . ."

"So, Tova, I'm happy because when a total stranger tells me to go screw myself, it means that for the first

time in thirteen years someone didn't see a poor disabled guy. She saw *me*." The weight of years lifted with
the revelation. "If a stranger in a nightclub interacts
with me as their equal, with no special treatment Tova,
it means I'm whole again."

Later, we met up with Dave, and my buddy and I
caught our flight back to L.A.

In the dark, I thought about the last time I traveled this route, when I first met Marcy. I thought about
Tova's question at the mojito bar: whether I was ready
for the future that increased mobility might make at-
tainable. For a patient kit, Bioness had shown survivors
use their new medical device; filmed me stroll along a
sandy beach with a friend. The company planned to
send the DVD to doctors and hospitals around the world
that wanted to see how the NESS could help survivors
of stroke and neurological disease walk again.

So I thought about Tova's anguish on her wedding day, and wondered whether I was ready to answer
the question she too confronted. I still didn't know if I
could follow my own advice to her when I unpacked next
morning in my old home with Marcy, and felt its memories, or later, after fresh driving lessons brought me to
another meeting at the Department of Motor Vehicles,
this one before Driver Safety Officer Vazquez.

This time, I'd answered every question on the
short written test correctly, down to a lucky guess as
to which type of vehicle was obliged to stop before it
could cross railroad tracks. Apparently ones filled with
hazardous chemicals must, a reminder that I was in
the section of the DMV reserved for truckers licensed
to haul loads, along with habitual DUIs. But when Ms.
Vazquez prepared to put me on the record, my doubts
erupted.

"Please," I raised a hand.

My hearing officer frowned at the interruption.

"Two examiners say I threatened pedestrians," I continued. "I don't know if it's right to try to put my life back together like this if I could hurt someone."

"The second examiner cleared you to try again," she countered.

"And if I fail a third test, it's over?"

"If a candidate can't satisfy three examiners, usually we tell them it's time to hang up their keys," she sighed. "But your instructor reports you safe to drive, and—"

"And I was safe to drive when I didn't see the pickup coming that killed my wife." The confession tumbled from my lips, the guilt of thirteen years that lay at the heart of Tova's question in San Francisco, and my doubts of whether I could follow my own advice to her.

"If I couldn't save my wife, why do I deserve another chance?"

"Because, Mr. Lewis, we all do," she said softly.

And then Erika Vazquez described what happened one night at her home, when her seven-year-old got a bad headache. How, as her daughter's pain grew, she called 911; watched helpless as medics ignored her desperate pleas for help, but instead followed protocol and investigated whether it was child abuse that led to a young girl's collapse on the kitchen floor by the time they arrived, and required referral to Child Protective Services. So instead of emergency patient evacuation, the paramedics questioned every person in the household, and filled paperwork until her stricken girl went into seizures. Erika told me how she insisted on riding with her daughter in the ambulance so as not to leave her side, and, with a pain that time might never soften, described the absence of urgency in the emergency room, as she stroked her girl's hand through a six-day coma until Erika was asked to complete one final form, and release her daughter from life support to her final place of rest. Her daughter was lost to a brain aneurysm, a heart attack of the brain, in which a caregiver's only hope is vigilance. Because when there's a change in the circulation within your head, every moment counts.

Erika told me how she found a way to her second chance; showed photos on the wall behind her desk of a new home, and a kind man with a daughter. She'd learned her own daughter's name, Stephanie, meant "crown," and she thought of her girl every day, crowned in heaven.

"It's your decision, Mr. Lewis, whether you want to try again," she said, as she brought my hearing to a close.

As we shook hands and I left the DMV that day, I knew, at last, the meaning of courage.

More driving lessons followed. Bryan showed me *Let's Go for a Drive*, a new DVD released by the Department of Motor Vehicles of mock tests given to teenagers who think they pass but don't, and the top ten reasons they fail. The DVD was likely unknown to millions of older drivers who, accident-free for decades, think they're safe to drive until three quick fails take them off the road for the rest of their lives; a DVD unseen by the population who would most benefit from the examiners' insights, which included that you could ask questions before your test began. And in October, when I met my examiner, this time at the DMV's Winnetka office for my last chance at a driver's license, I did.

"If I see a threat may I tell you, so you don't worry I haven't, and beat me to the brake?"

Harold looked startled, but he nodded assent and we were off, communication established as our test advanced, and we neared a busy intersection.

"I plan to slow and stop in case that woman with a stroller jaywalks," I maintained my narrative.

"No . . . go!" Harold called. "At these lights, we'll get stuck forever!"

So I accelerated through the corner, made some final turns, and passed the California driving test.

At the end of the month, the DMV issued an interim license, and to build my confidence without the safety net of instructor dual controls, Bryan recommended practice sessions in a regular car with my special prismatic glasses as final preparation for life on the roads of L.A.

It felt strange and wonderful to be behind the wheel with no more than Bryan's expert eyes to watch over me, my nerves stressed but controlled as we toured the San Fernando Valley in the midday sun, and I tested how to handle my car.

Toward the end of our hour, we were headed back home, and entered an intersection to make a left. We waited a long time for oncoming traffic to pass. The lights changed to yellow while I yielded to vehicles clear our intersection, then turned red. A northbound midnight blue Dodge remained, a hundred and fifty feet in the distance, as cross traffic moved forward on its green.

"Make the turn. Clear the intersection," Bryan ordered, terse as ever.

I was already on it, and scanned as Ken, then Bryan, had trained me through months of lessons. Which was why I saw the Dodge accelerate to over forty and run the red; why, for the first time in so many years I put the pedal to the metal. Full throttle, the sedan roared, its tires burned rubber, and with hand-over-hand steering, the car rocketed on target into the turn. And that was why the Dodge didn't impale Bryan, but instead hit inches behind our rear wheel and smashed into those car panels, ripping the back fender from the car frame, so it flew off into the intersection.

"My lights were green!" shouted the young driver, angry as she emerged unharmed from her car, and I felt no escape from the certainty of what would happen to the typed piece of paper in my pocket, my interim driver's license. With her version of events, my driving record, and only Bryan and myself—both interested parties—to contradict it, I didn't stand a chance. The DMV wouldn't issue a full license, they'd pull my interim one, and never let me drive again. But I no longer cared: I had saved Bryan's life, and nothing else mattered.

But witnesses began to gather, who saw the Dodge blow through the red. As the driver switched her story, to claim the lights were yellow when she entered the intersection, the witnesses became emphatic—that was still illegal. In fact, one said they saw her talking on her cell phone, oblivious to red lights and intersection alike, when she accelerated into Bryan and me.

"Mr. Lewis," Brenda Maples said next day, when I called to ask if she'd give her eyewitness account to the adjuster, "I never met you before, and know nothing about your past. But for five total strangers in L.A. to stop where they're going on a Friday at lunchtime, and come to your rescue, tells me one thing: You're protected by some very powerful karma."

CHAPTER TWENTY-TWO

CONFLUENCE

From amidst the darkness set sail
with the softness
Wind coming in picking up momentum
Cutting crisply through the thickness
Trailblazing through affliction
Dancing like a lion roaring rising
out of nothing

—Matisyahu,
"Aish Tamid"

In the summer of 2008, a happily married Tova visited us with her husband Jason and their baby girl. Born on Mother's Day, little Naomi giggled when I held her in my arms, full of a newborn's fresh life and joy. In the fall, there was a letter from my internist.

"Dear Simon, I am writing to let you know of an exciting change in my practice," began the letter from Dr. Brousseau, that signaled the start of the annual

health insurance ritual that once more would determine survival of the fittest. "Unfortunately," my doctor's letter continued, "economic realities do not allow
me to continue caring for patients with an HMO."

Maybe this year the business of caring had a new
tactic. Insurance was an evanescent mystery, impossible to keep up with, let alone understand, for Brousseau's clinic processed me as usual when I arrived, and
administered follow-up bone density and Holter tests.

I held my breath as I heard my internist approach my cubicle, ready for more bone loss and daily
medication to limit future fractures, as he entered, then
examined my results.

"There's marked improvement," Dr. Brousseau
noted instead with surprise, and showed me the printout. "Your pelvis's bone density has increased ten percent, and your spine by almost twenty."

"It's because I'm mobile again," I guessed.

"You should show this to the Bioness people," he
nodded. "It's very significant. At this point, Simon, your
bone loss is only mild."

A nurse handed him the new Holter results.

"Well, well . . . ," he murmured. "Your heart rate's
gone to an average sixty-five . . . and the longest pause
has dropped from three-and-a-half seconds to two."

"Is that good?" I asked.

"Yes," he replied simply, "it's much better than
last time."

"Do I still need to do a Holter every year?"

"Nope." He sounded both surprised and pleased.
"But we'll always keep an eye on it."

On the way home, this result felt more significant
than renewed strength in my bones, though I wasn't
sure why. But if the Holter showed improvement in
my heart, my nerve-blood circulation must have flowed
better now for over two years, the time Dr. Ahn said

it might take after I gave up my second rib to feel the full benefit. Then, something new entered my thoughts. You never notice gradual recovery, the kind you take for granted. I saw it only when I read back through notes I made for my book; a desperate one after my weekend with Tova and Jason two years before, of a climactic migraine and days of crushing pain that ended, "So many theories. So uncertain what each day will bring."

There was still no certainty what each new day would bring, but I realized that for each one since, I did feel . . . better. I remembered Dr. Collins, his cryptic farewell at UCLA that "all your problems are circulatory."

Perhaps along a hidden pathway, an unknown brain-heart connection gradually responded to the easier flow within me, and enabled the beat of my heart to flow, also. And in that moment, through my entire journey in search of answers, I understood what Dr. Collins meant. His words were the map to the hidden path that started with Western medicine, then led to Eastern philosophies and treatments, to Chinese medicine, and then to Dr. Zhong who spoke of "qi"—our one-life circulation. Now, as Castro and Ahn's releases allowed more of that life force to run through me, and the NESS channeled my nerve flow as I walked, I sensed how Collins was right; that the way to find and stay on the hidden path was to feel the current of that circulation every instant as it coursed through my life; to think more about the journey than the destination, and find the best line down the rapids and eddies, the best balance and calmest current. I saw how the improved flow slowly brought me to this, my simple epiphany: The hidden path to full recovery is the day-by-day choice of the best way to flow.

As the benefits Dr. Ahn promised continued, and my nerve-blood circulation rose, this became clearer to me. It brought something else, too: a strange revelation which brought full recovery for my soul through the insight that all my struggles since the hit-and-run that crushed my life made it no less sweet, in fact the opposite. Slowly and gently, they deepened my faith in the potential of each and every moment that remained, ever since I first saw light in the window of my room at ✓ Cedars. They drew me closer to the eternal flame of life and the joy of its warmth.

Perhaps it's the way of all nature, and recovery has the same enduring attraction for us as gravity does the planets, even when there are days when we feel as if the sun doesn't rise, because this is a warmth that comes from within, the spark in the center of our souls. In the whispering depths of heart and mind, I know that place in the mountains I entered in a coma, where consciousness ends and life starts anew that is always familiar, always interesting, and understand what it means to awaken each day in a world that is both. I remember when I bathed in the river of time and felt the moment when time became flat, discovered that everything is now. Whether it's the Roman Tiber, the Ganges, the Greek Styx, or the river Jordan, I know the river I hear, the one that whispers through each of us down from the mountain deep within, is the nerve-flow of life itself, the one circulation within us all.

I feel it so clearly now, so calmly, my soul within. I feel how the mind links all possibilities in every waking and sleeping moment, from the deep-stored race memory that stirred in my coma to a fourteen-year path ✓ I followed, to an answer that lets me savor the simple miracle each morning as night fades and the sun glides toward the horizon, pure gold, in the soft light before dawn. It's the answer to a question asked through the ages.

But where shall wisdom be found? and where is the place of understanding?

> *. . . The topaz of Ethiopia shall not equal it, neither shall it be valued with pure gold.*
> *Whence then cometh wisdom? and where is the place of understanding?*
> —Book of Job, 28:12–20

An eternal quest for faith, for the wisdom to understand and live with affliction, the words of the Old Testament beg for answers as powerfully now as two-and-a-half-thousand years ago when they were first written by an Israelite and attributed to Job, the "greatest of all the men of the east," who remained steadfast through his suffering. Timeless questions perhaps answered in the words of Moses, over a thousand years before:

> *For the Lord thy God bringeth thee into a good land, a land of brooks of water, of fountains and depths that spring out of valleys and hills;*
> *A land of wheat and barley, and vines and fig-trees and pomegranates; a land of oil olive and honey;*
> —Deuteronomy 8:7–8

Whether or not I could find all the answers to my afflictions, I'd found my Promised Land, my spiritual full recovery, a faith that will sustain the rest of my life. It lay in my now profound appreciation of the outcome of so many choices I can make, and peaceful acceptance of those I cannot. Full recovery on the hidden path is not only about choices you make, but also about what it means to find that a choice is forever taken away; about how much, exactly, still remains.

On my journey of discovery along the hidden
path, I'd reached that question and learned the answer,
understood what truly *remains*.

Asked since the dawn of human lineage, Job's
desperate questions looked for an answer to the plains
of Ethiopia where our history began, from where our
early ancestors migrated around the world. There were
probably about ten thousand of us in Africa back then,
and we're all descendants from that small band. We are,
each and every one of us, companions on our search for
a better tomorrow, all African, all distant cousins—one
people with identical roots. A shared heritage reflected
in the ancient words of Job, who was so much closer
than us to our distant past, and our race memory of the
"topaz of Ethiopia."

Every day for me is a fresh start, a new blessing,
for I understand the feelings first expressed by Job, and
made poetic by an unknown Confederate soldier; words
which link all who need to find the hidden path, across
the millennia:

A Creed for Those Who Have Suffered

I asked God for strength,
that I might achieve.
I was made weak,
that I might learn humbly to obey.
I asked for health,
that I might do great things.
I was given infirmity,
that I might do better things.
I asked for riches,
that I might be happy.
I was given poverty,
that I might be wise.
I asked for power,

that I might have the praise of men.
I was given weakness,
that I might feel the need of God.
I asked for all things that I might enjoy life.
I was given life,
that I might enjoy all things.
I got nothing I asked for,
but everything I had hoped for.
Almost despite myself,
my unspoken prayers were answered.
I am among men most richly blessed.

I understand the past need not limit the future, and when I make plans for mine, I remember some lyrics that offer the key to my soul that I sought for so long in the darkness. The song repeats the simple question that everyone in search of the hidden path for themselves or a loved one must answer each day to attain full recovery.

In December of 2008, my agent Steve submitted my manuscript to Santa Monica Press, and on March 2, 2009, fifteen years to the day after my hit-and-run accident, Jeffrey Goldman accepted it for his fall catalog, and publication in 2010.

I hope this book helps you find your way, so you don't regret the life that you knew yesterday has ended, but celebrate your life that begins today. So you open your eyes every morning, awake to the promise of life, the sunsets and sunrises that encircle us. My final song of full recovery, and the key question to which I found my answer is:

Will the day be warm and bright,
or will it snow?
There are people waiting here,
Who really want to know

Will the day be warm and bright,
or will it snow?
There are people waiting now
Who really have to know

—Caravan,
"Disassociation/100% Proof"

All of our hands and all of our voices link us all across time. Let the river of life run within you, and all your days be warm and bright. Rise and shine in good health, and may your God go with you.

ACKNOWLEDGMENTS

I'm forever grateful to the surgeons, doctors, nurses, and therapists who saved my life and whose peers are unsung heroes for so many. Almost as important to the existence of this book are the people who guided me toward its creation. I'm especially indebted to my agent Steve Wasserman for his unflagging determination that this book see the light of day; and my attorney, Eric Weissmann, who met me for lunch the day after I called, to resume our friendship after more than a decade as if without interruption, and his loyal team of Irma, Aida, and Anita.

I was blessed to find Santa Monica Press and its publisher Jeffrey Goldman, who always did what was best for my book. His copy editor, Breanna Murphy, spared me the embarrassment of grammatical and typographical errors, and his team brought the book to this final form, in which any remaining flaws are mine alone.

Good feedback helps, and I was lucky to receive it all the way through, first from my Aunt Zena, whose second home is the bookstores of Oxford, to writers and friends including Herbert Gold, Carolyn Hennesy, Bernard Lewis, Roy Lilley, and David Pryce-Jones.

Other supporters included Richard Jeffs, who connected me with Simon Clegg at Above the Title Productions in London to record an audiobook; friends and colleagues from USC, UCLA Extension, and Cambridge; Bill Graham, Jon Otworth, and Angel Urbina for the book website; and John Brainard, Marc Coury, Wayne Evans, Jennifer French, Harry Hyman, Marion Kukurudz, Joseph Leahy, John Lehner, Jim Presnal, David Roy, Ronnie Rubin, Andrew Solt, Charles Weiner, Terry Tegnazian, Scott Whittle, and Barry Wilson.

My final thanks are to my parents who brought me into this world twice, my two brothers, and their wives and children. Family, and the memory of who went before us, give meaning every day to life, full recovery, and tomorrow.

DISCLAIMER

Subject to the disclaimer below, names and descriptions of some of the less familiar medical terms and technologies appearing in this book are offered for readers, based on reference sources such as Wikipedia, and the author's experience of them. To see examples of some images online, readers are invited to explore www.riseandshinethebook.com

The statements in my book and on the website are based on my personal research and experiences as a patient, and are not intended and do not provide medical advice, diagnosis, cure, or treatment for any individual's physical problems or medical conditions. Do not rely on any information that you read in my book or the website (or obtain by posts, e-mails, or links to other websites) to replace advice from a qualified medical professional. Information in my book and on the website does not constitute an endorsement or claim for any product or service.

All postings on the website by third party contributors are the sole responsibility of the person who made such posting and we are not liable in any way for any

postings or any opinions expressed in them, including, but not limited to, for any errors or omissions in any postings.

GLOSSARY

405 freeway. A major north-south highway in Southern California.

ABC. The U.S. radio and TV network American Broadcasting Company; **KABC-TV** is the owned-and-operated flagship television station in Los Angeles of the American Broadcasting Company.

activities of daily living (ADLs). The ability or inability to perform these activities—which include feeding, bathing, dressing, grooming, work, homemaking, and leisure—are used by health professionals to measure functional status.

acupuncture. A technique of inserting and manipulating fine needles into specific points on the body to relieve pain or for therapeutic purposes, associated with **traditional Chinese medicine**.

AFO (ankle foot orthotic). An orthosis or brace, usually plastic, worn on the ankle joint and all or part of the foot. AFOs control position and motion of the ankle, compensate for weakness, or correct deformities. They control the ankle directly, and can be designed to control the knee joint indirectly as well.

aortogram. A radiographic record of the heart's aorta, resulting from aortography.

Arizona Dystonia Institute, Institute for Developmental Behavioral Neurology. The Scottsdale, Arizona examination, evaluation, and research clinic, led by its director, Drake D. Duane, MD, offers examinations and evaluations of diverse neurological disorders.

arthrogram. An X-ray of a joint after injection of a contrast medium or dye.

Babinski's reflex. The extension of the toes upward when the sole of the foot is stroked firmly on the outer side from the heel to the front; normal in infants under the age of two years but an indication of brain or spinal cord injury in older persons.

baby butterfly needle. A twenty-one- to twenty-five-gauge needle, with two plastic "wings" on either side. The needle is held by the "wings" and placed into the vein, generally at a fairly shallow angle. The "wings" allow the phlebotomist to grasp the needle very close to the end, to ensure accuracy.

Blake, William. The English poet, painter, and printmaker.

botulinum toxin (Botox). A medication and a neurotoxic protein produced by the bacterium Clostridium botulinum. It is sold commercially under brand names including Botox, and used in minute doses to treat muscle spasms and in cosmetic applications.

brain-mapping program. A set of neuroscience techniques conceived as a higher form of neuro-imaging, to produce brain images supplemented by other data analysis to yield maps, which project measures of behavior onto brain regions.

Brokaw, Tom. The American television journalist and author, best known as former anchor and managing editor of NBC Nightly News.

Chamberlain, Wilt. The American professional NBA basketball player. The 7-foot-1-inch Chamberlain weighed 250 lbs. as a rookie, before bulking up to 275 lbs. and, eventually, over 300 lbs. with the Los Angeles Lakers.

choline, also **phosphatidylcholine (PC).** A nutritional supplement used for its suggested advantages to liver function and as a nutrient for brain function.

Christ's College, Cambridge University. The school where the author was an undergraduate.

Code Blue. The hospital emergency code used to convey, with efficiency and without alarm, that a patient requires immediate resuscitation, most often as the result of cardiac arrest.

computer-enhanced graphics (CEG). Used in the book to describe advanced differential diagnosis of the jaw, head, and neck, CEG employs multiple data processes to build graphical representations to evaluate, diagnose, treat, and measure patient outcome.

cone beam CT (CBCT). A three-dimensional cone beam computed tomography that produces high-resolution X-ray images (tomographs) for detailed evaluation of the mandible.

CPR (cardio pulmonary resuscitation). The combination of chest compressions and mouth-to-
mouth breathing used when breathing, heartbeat, or both, stop.

cranioplasty. The surgical repair of defect or deformity of the skull.

CT pelvis, 3-D reconstruction. An additional technique that assembles CT images into a three-dimensional display of the pelvis.

CT scan (computed tomography scan). An X-ray
procedure that uses the aid of a computer to create a series of detailed pictures of areas inside
the body in a single plane.

debridement. The removal of a patient's dead, damaged, or infected tissue to improve healing potential of the remaining healthy tissue.

defibrillator. An electronic device that administers
electric shock of preset voltage to the heart
through the chest wall, in an attempt to restore
normal rhythm of the heart during ventricular
fibrillation.

dystonia. A neurological disorder with variable symptoms that reflect sustained involuntary muscle contraction, the causes of which are not yet
known or understood.

edema. An abnormal accumulation of fluid beneath the
skin, or in one or more cavities of the body.

El Dorado. The mythical city of gold, a legend that
originated in sixteenth-century South America.

electrocardiography (ECG or EKG). A transtho-
racic interpretation of the electrical activity of

the heart over time captured and externally recorded by skin electrodes.

electroencephalography (EEG). The recording of electrical activity along the scalp produced by the firing of neurons within the brain.

electrognathography (EGN), jaw tracking computer tests and analyses. Measures and records mandibular movement using a jaw tracking sensor array. Three dimensions of movement can be measured: vertical, anterior/posterior, and lateral.

electromyography (EMG). The science of recording the electrical activity of muscle fibers, in general either surface or needle (intramuscular) EMG. Each electrode track gives only a very local picture of the activity of the whole muscle, but bilateral, simultaneous measurement of the craniomandibular muscles can be recorded.

endodontist. A dentist who specializes in matters concerning the inside of the tooth, namely the tooth pulp, which is comprised of nerve tissue and blood vessels.

existentialism. The work of nineteenth- and twentieth-century philosophers who took the human subject—the acting, feeling, living human individual and his or her conditions of existence—as a starting point for philosophical thought.

FDA. The U.S. Food and Drug Administration, responsible for protection and promotion of American health through inspection, education, and enforcement of matters including food, drugs, and medical devices.

F-Scan. A measurement system that captures dynamic

in-shoe pressure information revealing interaction between foot and footwear.

Galium-Heel. A blend of several homeopathic remedies used for suggested advantages to the immune system and to combat viral infections.

Gelsemium Homaccord. A homeopathic medication used for suggested advantages to recurrent, occipital headache, stiff neck, and upper back neuralgia.

heart arrhythmia. An irregular heartbeat with symptoms including palpitations, dizziness, fainting, shortness of breath, and chest discomfort.

herbal tea. A part of **traditional Chinese medicine**; includes more than three hundred herbs commonly used today, with a history of use that goes back at least two thousand years.

HIPAA. The Health Insurance Portability and Accountability Act enacted by the U.S. Congress in 1996.

Holter monitor. A portable device for continuously monitoring electrical activity of the central nervous system for at least twenty-four hours. The most common use is for monitoring the heart, but can also be used for monitoring **EEG**.

homeostasis. The property of a system, such as the human body, which regulates its internal environment and tends to maintain a stable, constant condition.

Huntington, The. A private, nonprofit institution consisting of the Huntington Library, Art Collections and Botanical Gardens. It is located in San Marino near Pasadena, northeast of downtown Los Angeles.

hyperbaric chamber, or **hyperbaric medicine.** A medical use of oxygen at a level higher-than-atmospheric pressure.

intra-oral orthotic. A removable device that fits over the teeth in one arch, to guide mandible into new position, in which teeth hold the jaw in correct balance and alignment.

Jackson-Pratt drain. A rubber tube with squeeze bulb at one end, the other inserted into body, to remove excess fluid that can collect after surgery.

Jaws of Life. The hydraulic tools used by emergency rescue personnel to assist in vehicle extrication of crash victims, and for rescues from other small spaces. The tools include cutters, spreaders, and rams.

Jewish Federation. The confederation of Jewish social agencies, volunteer programs, educational bodies, and related organizations found within most cities in North America that host a Jewish community.

JVA (joint vibration analysis). An electronic recording and computer-enhanced examination and interpretation of joint vibrations (tissue pressure waves in the jaw).

Lake Tahoe. A large freshwater lake in the Sierra Nevadas located along the border between California and Nevada, and major tourist attraction for both states.

Lee, Peggy. The singer with Benny Goodman's band, known for her sex appeal and sultry tunes, who was given a Lifetime Achievement Grammy in 1995.

Leibinger miniplates. Titanium implants used during craniotomy to correct large skull defects and fractures.

Let's Go for a Drive. A DVD released by the California Department of Motor Vehicles.

Long Beach Harbor. Located about twenty miles South of Los Angeles, on the Pacific Coast.

Lucasfilm Foundation. The private foundation of acclaimed filmmaker George Lucas, creator of *Star Wars, Indiana Jones,* and many other blockbuster films.

Lymphomyosot. A homeopathic drug used for suggested advantages to tissue edema and swelling.

Magic Mountain. The Six Flags Magic Mountain amusement park with roller coasters, games and attractions just north of Los Angeles.

mandible. The lower jawbone that holds lower teeth in place.

maxillofacial surgery. A recognized international surgical specialty; surgery to correct a wide spectrum of diseases, injuries and defects in the head, neck, face, jaws, and the hard and soft tissues of the oral and maxillofacial region.

moxibustion. A therapy of **traditional Chinese medicine** using moxa, or mugwort. Ground up into a fluff, practitioners can burn the fluff indirectly, with **acupuncture** needles, or sometimes burn it on a patient's skin.

MRI, MRA, and **MRV.** A two- and three-dimensional image reconstruction with applications including evaluation and diagnosis of **thoracic outlet syndrome (TOS).**

MRN (magnetic resonance neurogram). A diagnostic utility in surgical treatment of peripheral nerve disorders.

Munch, Edvard. The Norwegian Symbolist painter. *The Scream* is his best-known composition.

Music Center, Performing Arts Center of Los Angeles County. Located in downtown Los Angeles, the Music Center is comprised of four venues: the Walt Disney Concert Hall, the Dorothy Chandler Pavilion, the Ahmanson Theatre, and the Mark Taper Forum, as well as outdoor theaters, plazas, and gardens.

Narcissus. The Greek mythological hero whose divine punishment was to fall in love with a reflection in a pool, not realizing it was his own, and perish there, not able to leave the beauty of his own reflection.

nerve block. A procedure that relieves pain by interrupting how pain signals are sent to the brain, usually by injecting a substance into or around a nerve, or into the spine.

orthotic. An orthopedic appliance designed to support, straighten, or improve functioning of a body part. (See **intra-oral orthotic**.)

osteomyelitis. An infection of bone or bone marrow with a propensity for progression, usually caused by bacteria.

panorex. A panoramic X-ray of the jaw that shows full views of upper and lower jaws, teeth, and surrounding structures.

PDNs (private duty nurses). Professional practitioners who give direct, comprehensive care on an hourly or live-in basis.

piriformis The muscle that originates in front of the sacrum (upper part of the pelvis).

qi. In **traditional Chinese medicine**, an active principle forming part of any living thing, often translated as "energy flow."

rads. A unit used to measure energy absorbed by a material from radiation.

resection. In surgery, the removal of part or whole of an organ or other bodily structure.

ribectomy. The resection of a rib.

San Fernando Valley. The area to the north of Los Angeles with many residential communities.

scoliosis. A medical condition in which person's spine is curved from side to side, shaped like an "s," and may also be rotated.

SPECT (single photon emission computed tomography) brain scan. A nuclear medicine tomographic imaging technique using gamma rays, able to provide functional, 3-D information.

spinal myelogram. A procedure that involves injecting a radio-opaque dye into the spinal canal and taking X-ray pictures of the dye. Because of the dangers associated with this procedure, it is usually only performed when a surgeon intends to operate and wants an accurate idea of the sort of damage that may exist in the spine.

SPLATT (split anterior tibial tendon transfer). Used for treatment of equinovarus deformity of the foot.

Tae Kwon Do. One of the world's most popular martial arts in terms of the number of practitioners, and the national sport of South Korea.

Tantalus. The Greek mythological figure whose punishment, now proverbial for temptation without satisfaction (the source of the word *"tantalize"*), was to stand in a pool of water beneath a fruit tree with low branches. Whenever he reached for the fruit, the branches raised his intended meal from his grasp. Whenever he bent down to get a drink, the water receded before he could get any. Over his head towered a threatening stone.

temporomandibular joint (jaw). Connects mandible to the skull. Disorder and resultant disease and dysfunction (TMJD, TMJ, or TMD) can result in significant pain and impairment.

Three Fates. In Greek mythology, our destiny depended on three sisters depicted seated at a spinning wheel, where they spun the thread of our existence and determined our futures. The one continuous skein of silk was woven by Clotho, measured by Lachesis, until finally, in a very literal sense, cut short by the shears of Atropos.

tomographs. Detailed X-ray images of tissue structure lying in a predetermined plane, while blurring or eliminating detail in images of structures in other planes; used to study movement of the mandible.

TOS (thoracic outlet syndrome). A group of disorders involving compression at the superior thoracic outlet which affect the brachial plexus (nerves that pass into the arms from the neck), and/or the subclavian artery and vein (blood vessels that pass between the chest and upper extremity).

traditional Chinese medicine (TCM). A range of tra

ditional medical practices based on observations of nature, the cosmos, our human body, and *qi*. Although well accepted in the mainstream of medical care throughout East Asia, it is considered an alternative medical system in much of the Western world, and includes a broad array of treatments such as **acupuncture** with **moxibustion**, herbal medicine, diet therapy, and massage.

Traumeel. A homeopathic combination medication used for suggested advantages to injuries, wounds, pain, bleeding, muscle tone, and antiviral effect.

UCLA Extension The University of California, Los Angeles continuing education division designed to meet the needs of adults of all ages.

USC School of Cinematic Arts. The University of Southern California's center for the creation, study, research, and development of cinema, television, and interactive media, which confers degrees ranging from bachelor's to doctorate levels.

Valhalla. In Norse mythology, an enormous, majestic hall ruled over by the god Odin.

Van Nuys. A district in the San Fernando Valley in Los Angeles.

Victims of Crime Program, California. A program to assist injured victims of crime with otherwise uninsured expenses.

Wachovia Securities. Now Wells Fargo Advisors.

Weirdstone of Brisingamen, The. A fantasy story by the English author Alan Garner, first published in 1960.

West Traffic Division. The Los Angeles Police Department division responsible for investigation of traffic collisions and traffic related crimes for its Operations-West Bureau

WGA, Writers Guild of America West. A labor union that represents thousands of writers, including those of TV shows, movies, news programs, documentaries, animation, and new media.

Xanadu. A place appearing in Samuel Taylor Coleridge's poem *Kubla Khan*, where Kubla Khan "did/A stately pleasure-dome decree."

Z-plasty. A plastic surgery technique that is used to improve the functional and cosmetic appearance of scars.

RESOURCES

STROKE

American Stroke Association, a division of American
Heart Association, and *Stroke Connection* magazine
(800) AHA-USA1 (242-8721); www.americanheart.org

National Stroke Association
(800) STROKES (787-6537); www.stroke.org

National Institute of Neurological Disorders and Stroke
www.ninds.nih.gov

BRAIN INJURY

Brain Injury Association of America
(800) 444-6443; www.biausa.org

SPINAL CORD INJURY

National Spinal Cord Injury Association
(800) 962-9629; http://www.spinalcord.org

INSURANCE

Medicare
(800) 633-4227; www.medicare.gov

California Heath Insurance Counseling and Advocacy
Program (HICAP)
(800) 434-0222

VICTIM COMPENSATION PROGRAMS

U.S. Department of Justice, Victims of Crime Act
(VOCA) Assistance and Compensation Programs
http://www.ojp.usdoj.gov/ovc/help/links.htm

State Level: National Association of Crime Victim
Compensation Boards
http://www.nacvcb.org

California Victim Compensation Program
(800) 777-9229; www.vcgcb.ca.gov

FICTIONALIZED NAMES

The names of some doctors, clinicians, nurses and patients involved in my story, including the following, have been fictionalized, because the individuals were either untraceable or requested privacy. Accordingly, any resemblance between any individuals with these names, and actual events locales or persons, living or dead, depicted in this book, is entirely coincidental:

Almendros
Anderson, Phil
Avidan
Banning, Michelle
Coulton
Croft, John
Endiman, Casper
Flores, Julian
Kern, Bruce
Kingsley, Ann
Koster
Neame, Mark and Ruth
Polk
Ramsay

Rose
Rossi, Pauline
Sloane, Alan
Stein, Norman
Stewart, Henry
Stone
Terrill, Frank
Thomason
Turner, Sally
Whitney
Whittaker

Ben, Bergen family, Beryl, Beth, Carol, Connie, Erica,
Gloria, Hank, Harold, Harvey, Karin, Lloyd, Luke,
Marka, Mary, Melissa, Nancy, Pete, Roy, Ted, Tim,
Tina, Viktor, Zack

INDEX

A Creed for Those Who Have Suffered, 326

activities of daily living, 79

acupressure. *See under* Eastern medicine

acupuncture. *See under* Eastern medicine

AFO (ankle foot orthotic), 131, 140, 228

Age Old Friends (film), 61, 111

Alfred Mann Foundation, 287, 300

    Ben (fictionalized), 288, 289, 290

    See also Byers, Chuck; implantable bionic technologies; Mann, Alfred

aneurysm, 114, 317

aortogram, 25

Arizona Dystonia Institute, 181, 242, 294

arthrogram, 216

Babinski's reflex, 125, 214

baby butterfly needle, 157

biomechanics, 194, 275

Bioness, 290, 297, 298, 299, 300, 301, 315, 322. *See also* NESS; Ulrich, Steven

BIONS, 287, 288

BioResearch conference, 274

Blake, William, 88

bone density, 322

Book of Job, 325

Botox, 181, 182, 294, 295

brace, 131, 137, 165, 228, 275, 288. *See also* AFO (ankle foot orthotic)

brain-mapping program, 124

Brokaw, Tom, 22

Buspar, 87, 89

Burrage, Bryan, 309, 310, 317, 318, 319. *See also* DMV

Byers, Chuck, 287, 289, 290. *See also* Alfred Mann Foundation

California Victims of Crime Program, 200, 202, 205, 282, 348

Cambridge University, 120, 121, 129, 235, 265

Casa Colina Rehabilitation Center, 298, 299, 301, 303, 307. *See also* Hanson, Mathu

Cedars-Sinai Medical Center, 18, 19, 20, 22, 23, 25, 26, 35, 43, 45, 51, 53, 55, 57, 58, 73, 81, 83, 84, 88, 92, 95, 96, 98, 99, 101, 102, 103, 106, 107, 109, 110, 111, 112, 114, 115, 118, 121, 122, 123, 126, 127, 129, 130, 132, 140, 142, 148, 149, 150, 152, 153, 157, 158, 167, 168, 169, 181, 182, 183, 186, 188, 194, 195, 200, 207, 211, 212, 228, 284, 285, 289, 291, 296, 297, 324

Chamberlain, Wilt, 133

chemotherapy, 210

Chocolate War, The (film), 59

choline. *See under* homeopathic medicine

circulation, 20, 178, 179, 186, 246, 256, 258, 274, 280, 281, 282, 317, 322, 323, 324

COBRA. *See under* health insurance

Code Blue, 89, 90

cognitive retraining, 139

Coleman, Ken, 293, 301, 302, 318. *See also* Driver Preparation program

coma, 34–35, 37–39, 41–45, 80, 316

comascape, 34–35, 37–39, 41–45, 61, 104, 185

computer-enhanced graphics, 194

conditioning protocol, 299

cone beam CT, 194. *See also* CT scan

Continuing Disability Review. *See under* social security

contrecoup, 103

coup, 103

CPR, 16, 18

craniomandibular system, 194

cranioplasty, 145

craniosacral massage, 227

craniotomy, 29

"crash," 173, 189, 200, 203, 205, 219, 220, 227, 236, 237, 238, 241, 243, 247, 255, 256, 259, 284

CT scan, 145, 152, 170, 171, 194, 208, 209, 255, 258

Day of Atonement, 297

Deal or No Deal (television show), 284. *See also* Mandel, Howie

debridement, 130, 132

defibrillator, 89

Deuteronomy, 325

developmental optometry, 105, 137

DMV, 122, 286, 291, 301, 302, 303, 308, 309, 310, 315, 317–318, 319

DMV's Safety Office, 291, 315–317

Gloria (fictionalized), 309, 310

Harold (fictionalized), 317–318

Harvey (fictionalized), 301, 302, 308

Let's Go for a Drive (DVD), 317

See also Burrage, Bryan; Vazquez, Erika

Doctor Feelbad, 141, 278

Doctor Feelgood, 129, 134, 140, 149, 211, 212, 230, 232, 263, 264, 268, 271, 277, 278

Doctor Pelvis. *See* doctors: Johnson, Eric

Doctor Red Dots, 147-148, 187, 192

Doctor Together, 255, 258, 262

doctors

Ahn, Sam, 254, 255, 256, 257, 259, 262, 268, 269, 272, 274, 276, 277, 278, 279, 280, 281, 292, 322, 323 (*see also* Gonda Vascular Center)

Almendros (fictionalized), 86–87

Anderson, Phil (fictionalized), 19, 41, 78, 96, 126, 127, 130, 131, 195

Avidan (fictionalized), 131

Banning, Michelle fictionalized), 150, 151, 154, 156, 157, 175, 202

Berman, Andrew, 183, 186, 187

Bersohn, 223, 230, 264, 269, 270, 271

Birnbaum, 125, 132

Brien, 27, 28, 40, 41, 104, 132, 133, 136, 141, 211

Brodney, Alan, 97, 105, 138, 139, 170, 284

Brousseau, Michael, 241, 255, 259, 269, 270, 292, 293, 321, 322

Castro, Daniel, 258, 259, 261, 262, 263, 265, 266, 267, 268, 274, 279

Collins, James, 244, 245, 246, 247, 248, 249, 250, 251, 252, 253, 254, 255, 256, 258, 263, 269, 295, 296, 323

Coulton (fictionalized), 76, 77, 79, 80, 97

Croft, John (fictionalized), 74, 77, 90, 92, 95, 228

Duane, Drake, 181, 182 (*see also* Arizona Dystonia Institute)

Endiman, Casper (fictionalized), 217, 218, 219, 229, 259, 261, 262, 275, 276, 292, 293, 294, 295, 296

Filler, Aaron, 215, 216, 217, 218, 219, 220, 221, 224, 226, 227, 228, 229, 230, 231, 232, 233, 234, 235, 236, 238, 239, 241, 242, 243, 246, 253, 258, 265

Flores, Julian (fictionalized), 214, 215, 216

Hershman, 207

Johnson, Eric, 207, 208, 209, 210, 211, 212, 213, 214, 229, 257

Kern, Bruce
(fictionalized), 25, 28, 29,
30, 45, 124, 144, 170, 171

Klapper, Robert, 132,
133, 135, 140, 141, 143,
148, 150, 159, 160, 167,
168, 169, 172, 174, 175,
178, 183, 202, 208, 210,
211, 229, 234

Bibi, 133, 150, 168

Mark, 133, 150

Koster (fictionalized),
264, 270

McBride, Duncan, 225

McKay, Duane, 193, 194,
195, 196, 199, 200, 203,
204, 205, 233, 274, 275,
282, 283, 301

Joanna, 205, 233

Rudy, 205

Moreland, 206, 207

Neame, Mark
(fictionalized), 22, 24, 26,
28, 51, 85

Polk (fictionalized), 165,
166, 178 (see also Rancho
Los Amigos Medical
Center)

Provda, Lois, 138, 139,
159, 167, 174, 175, 181,
186, 188, 189, 190, 192,
206, 214, 239

Ramsay (fictionalized),
25, 30, 31

Rose (fictionalized), 145,
146

Saxton, Ernestina, 236,
237, 238, 239, 240, 241,
242, 245, 248, 249, 253,
254, 255, 257, 258, 259,
268, 271, 277, 295, 296

Seeger, 208, 216

Shelton, 157, 158, 172,
173

Skaggs, Barry, 187, 191,
192, 193

Sloane, Alan
(fictionalized), 27, 41

Stein, Norman
(fictionalized), 84

Stewart, Henry
(fictionalized), 144, 145,
148, 151, 152, 154, 167,
168, 169, 170, 171, 177,
178, 185, 227

Stone (fictionalized), 214,
216, 217, 218, 222, 240

Terrill, Frank
(fictionalized), 43, 123,
133

Thomason (fictionalized),
235, 237, 238

Trachtenberg, George,
275, 280, 301, 303, 305

Turner, Sally
(fictionalized), 114,
120, 136 (see also TGIC
outpatient program)

Van Allan, Richard, 24,
25, 26, 99

Voight, 97, 99

Whitney (fictionalized),
103, 104, 106, 107, 188,
296

Whittaker (fictionalized),
147, 151, 156, 208, 209

Zhong, Shangyou, 178,
179, 180, 181, 202, 246,
263, 323 (see also Eastern
medicine)

"Dracula eye," 105, 123, 130,

132, 159, 170, 178, 185,
Driver Preparation program,
293, 308. *See also* Coleman,
Ken; Northridge Hospital;
San Marco, Gayle

dura, 24

dystonia, 182. *See also*
Arizona Dystonia Institute

Eastern medicine
  acupressure, 179, 189,
  227
  acupuncture, 178, 179,
  180, 189,
  herbal tea, 178, 189, 263
  moxibustion, 179
  qi, 180, 246, 323
  yoga, 200–202
  See also homeopathic
  medicine

edema, 255

EEG, 31, 33, 157, 182

EKG, 269, 304

El Dorado. *See under*
mythology

EMG, 83, 84, 151, 152, 157,
165, 182, 234, 294, 295

endodontist, 125

existentialism, 65

FDA, 290, 291, 294, 296, 297,
298

F-Scan, 304

functional stimulation. *See*
NESS

gait studio, 304. *See also*

doctors: Trachtenberg,
George

Galium-Heel. *See under*
homeopathic medicine

garbage anesthetic, 268, 271,
273, 277, 279. *See also* Doctor
Feelgood

Genesis, 47

Gelsemium Homaccord. *See
under* homeopathic medicine

genome, 9, 11, 60

Glasgow Coma Scale, 45, 49,
65

Gonda Vascular Center, 255.
See also doctors: Ahn, Sam;
UCLA Medical Center

Gordon, Keith, 21, 59, 82. See
also *Mother Night*; *Chocolate
War, The*

Great-West. *See under* health
insurance

gross incisions, 183

Hamlet (film), 152–154

hamsa, 313

Hanson, Mathu, 298,
299, 300, 301, 303, 307,
308. *See also* Casa Colina
Rehabilitation Center

health insurance
  COBRA, 52
  Great-West, 51, 52, 53,
  54, 55, 56, 96, 106, 110,
  111, 123, 131, 137, 193,
  196, 197
  health insurance
  portability, 196, 241
  Health Net, 196, 199,
  204, 207, 235, 240, 241

HIPAA, 172, 174, 196, 241

Kingsley, Ann (fictionalized), 242, 259

Medicare, 174, 175, 203, 222, 239, 240, 241, 259, 266, 282, 348

risk management, 52

Rossi, Pauline (fictionalized), 53, 54, 96, 106, 107, 123

WritersCare, 196, 197, 202, 207, 235

Health Net. *See under* health insurance

heart arrhythmia, 280

hematomas

epidural, 24, 231

subdural, 24

intracerebral, 24

herbal tea. *See under* Eastern medicine

heterotopic ossification, 209

HIPAA. *See under* health insurance

hit-and-run, 7, 15, 18, 37, 51, 82, 115, 200, 318, 324, 327

Hobson's choice, 235

Holter monitor, 230, 269, 270, 292, 293, 322

homeopathic medicine

choline, 182

Galium-Heel, 151

Gelsemium Homaccord, 151

Lymphomyosot, 151

Traumeel, 151

See also Eastern medicine

homeostasis, 30

Howie from Maui (HBO special). *See* Mandel, Howie

Huntington, The, 122

hyperbaric oxygen, 184, 253

implantable bionic technologies, 287. *See also* Alfred Mann Foundation

Indiana Jones (films), 180, 193

interventional radiology, 23–24. *See also* doctors: Van Allan, Richard

intra-oral orthotic, 195

Irving, David, 265, 303

Jackson-Pratt drain, 273

jaw, 24, 41, 78, 125, 127, 178, 187, 191, 194, 195, 200, 204, 205, 274, 283

Jaws of Life, 18, 19

Jewish Federation, 284

joint vibration analysis, 194, 205

karma, 319

Kingsley, Ann (fictionalized). *See under* health insurance

Klein, Patricia, 110, 112, 117. *See also* TGIC outpatient program

Kol Nidre, 297

Kubla Khan, 218

L.A. Times, 209

Lake Tahoe, 13

Lee, Peggy (singer), 95, 126

Leibinger miniplate, 168

Lloyd (fictionalized), 184. *See also* hyperbaric oxygen

Long Beach Harbor, 118

Look Who's Talking (film), 60, 155

Lucasfilm Foundation, 282

Mad Song (film), 208

Magic Mountain, 13

Mandel, Howie, 81, 105, 284

Mann, Alfred, 300. *See also* Alfred Mann Foundation

Markarian, Jean, 113, 114, 117, 136, 137. *See also* TGIC outpatient program

Mark Taper Forum, 40. *See also* Music Center, Performing Arts Center of Los Angeles County

Master Kim, 151, 154, 155, 156, 174, 200, 201, 202, 208, 281, 282. *See also* physical therapy; Tae Kwon Do

maxillofacial surgery, 187. *See also* doctors: Skaggs, Barry

Medicare. *See under* health insurance

microstimulator. *See* BIONS

migraine, 10, 242, 243, 244, 247, 248, 323. *See also* doctor: Collins, James; doctor: Saxton, Ernestina

Mother Night (film), 18, 21, 36, 82

motor strip, 158

Monty Python, 72

moxibustion. *See under* Eastern medicine

MRA, 245, 247, 249, 252, 254

MRI, 76, 148, 150, 158, 172, 173, 181, 184, 214, 216, 220, 221, 245, 246, 249, 252. *See also* neurogram

Music Center, Performing Arts Center of Los Angeles County, 13, 36, 40, 51, 52, 122, 174. *See also* Mark Taper Forum

mythology
   El Dorado, 10
   Narcissus, 121
   Tantalus, 226
   Three Fates, 163
   Valhalla, 34

Narcissus. *See under* mythology

nausea, 213, 273

Neame, Ruth (fictionalized), 22. *See also* doctors: Neame, Mark

nerve block, 217, 218, 220, 229, 254, 259, 261, 262, 263, 275

NESS, 288, 289, 290, 294, 296, 297, 298, 299, 300, 301, 303, 304, 305, 307, 308, 311, 313, 315, 323. *See also* Bioness

Neurobehavioral Status Exam, 139. *See also* doctors: Provda, Lois

neurogram, 220, 224, 229. *See also* MRI

No Exit (play). *See* existentialism

Northridge Hospital, 109–111, 122, 293, 303, 308

nuclear radiology. *See* doctors: Shelton, David

nurses

Connie (fictionalized), 184, 273

Karin (fictionalized), 57, 58, 59, 68, 70, 75, 91

Marka (fictionalized), 57, 58, 67, 68, 70, 75, 76, 78, 85

Melissa (fictionalized), 57, 58, 67, 68, 70, 72, 75, 78, 79

Roy (fictionalized), 57, 66

Tamara (fictionalized), 57, 62, 65, 66

Viktor (fictionalized), 224, 225, 226

opacity, 258

opioid, 272

orthotic, 195, 301, 305. *See also* AFO (ankle foot orthotic); intra-oral orthotic

osteomyelitis, 127, 131

Outpatient Driving and Vision Program, 285

Erica (fictionalized), 285, 286

Hank (fictionalized), 285, 286, 291

See also Cedars-Sinai Medical Center

panic attack, 228, 236, 280

panorex, 127

PDN (private duty nurse), 42, 52, 53, 54, 57, 62

pelvis, 24, 42, 75, 86, 104, 131, 136, 141, 146, 156, 158, 159, 166, 206, 207, 209, 300, 308, 322

Phantom Tollbooth, The, 203

physical therapy

Emily, 122, 134 (*see also* Northridge Hospital)

Luke (fictionalized), 75, 79, 98, 102 (*see also* Cedars-Sinai Medical Center)

therapists' 0–5 scale, 300

Tina (fictionalized), 84, 85, 86, 87, 88, 89, 91, 95, 98, 102 (*see also* Cedars-Sinai Medical Center)

Wilkinson, Joyce, 227 (*see also* UCLA Medical Center)

See also Tae Kwon Do; TGIC outpatient program; yoga

piriformis, 215, 221, 228, 229, 231, 254

Pollard, Stu, 217, 281. *See also* USC

prismatic glasses, 318

Provigil, 294, 296

qi. *See under* Eastern medicine

Rancho Los Amigos Medical Center, 161, 163, 164, 289, 294

Rancho Los Amigos Scale, 45, 99

resection, 135. *See also* ribectomy

ribectomy, 262, 270, 276, 278

Rossi, Pauline (fictionalized). *See under* health insurance

Roy, David, 134, 208. See also *Mad Song*

Russian Ark (film), 39

San Fernando Valley, 102, 147, 192, 318

San Marco, Gayle, 293, 301, 308. *See also* Driver Preparation program

Sartre, Jean-Paul. *See* existentialism

sciatic nerve, 159, 231

scoliosis, 244

sensory cortex, 288

sick sinus syndrome, 223, 264

Simon's Night (book), 98

sinus, 255, 258, 262, 265, 268

Sirens of Titan (book), 18

social security
    Continuing Disability Review, 203, 266
    Medicare (*see under* health insurance)

SPECT scan, 157, 159, 167, 172, 173, 179

spinal headache, 154

spinal myelogram, 152

spinal tap, 152, 157,

SPLATT, 145, 165

Star Wars (films), 239

stroke, 7–9, 69, 81, 110, 119, 125, 139, 151, 288, 294, 299,

315. *See also* TBI (traumatic brain injury)

Tae Kwon Do, 151, 154, 156, 190, 200
    hyung, 155
    See also Master Kim; physical therapy

Tantalus. *See under* mythology

TBI (traumatic brain injury), 7, 18, 20, 45, 58, 69, 70, 73, 76, 80, 98, 124, 138, 139, 145, 149, 158, 165, 184, 188, 209, 210, 214, 293, 294. *See also* stroke

TED hose, 224

tendon transfer, 165, 175, 182, 294

TGIC outpatient program, 110, 112, 113, 114, 116, 117, 119, 120, 122, 123, 125, 129, 131, 132, 136, 137, 142, 293
    Carol (fictionalized), 114, 118
    Chris, 114–115
    Flaherty, Debra, 110
    Ola, 111, 112, 118, 119, 293
    Pete (fictionalized), 114, 118, 119
    Ted (fictionalized), 114, 118, 119
    Zack (fictionalized), 115, 118, 141
    See also doctors: Turner, Sally (fictionalized); Klein, Patricia; Markarian, Jean; Northridge Hospital; physical therapy

thoracic outlet syndrome (TOS), 214, 252, 253, 255, 268, 340

Three Fates. *See under* mythology

TOS. *See* thoracic outlet syndrome

tomography, 205. *See also* SPECT scan; CT scan

Tova, 39, 40, 82, 254, 255, 283, 284, 308, 310, 311, 312, 313, 314, 315, 316, 321, 323

traditional Chinese medicine. *See* Eastern medicine

traumatic brain injury. *See* TBI

UCLA Extension, 82

UCLA Medical Center, 207, 208, 211, 213, 214, 215, 219, 227, 230, 238, 239, 242, 244, 255, 263, 269, 277, 295, 323

Ulrich, Steven, 298. *See also* Bioness

USC (University of Southern California), 14, 21, 136, 217, 282

Valhalla. *See under* mythology

Van Nuys, 200

vascular surgery. *See* doctors: Ahn, Sam

Vazquez, Erika, 315, 316. *See also* DMV

ventriculostomy, 25

Wailing Wall, 31

Warren, Harvey and Joy, 16, 37, 157

Weide, Bob, 21, 36, 82. *See also Mother Night*

Weirdstone of Brisingamen, The, 120

Weissmann, Eric, 293

West Traffic Division, 21

Wind in the Willows, The, 60

Wizard of Oz, The, 220

Writers Guild of America, 196

WritersCare. *See under* health insurance

Xanadu. See *Kubla Khan*

yoga. *See under* Eastern medicine

Zanaflex, 218

Z-plasty, 183. *See also* doctors: Berman, Andrew